Functional Remediation for Bipolar Disorder

Functional Remediation for Bipolar Disorder

Eduard Vieta

Director, Bipolar Disorders Program, Clinical Institute of Neuroscience,
Hospital Clinic of Barcelona;
Professor of Psychiatry,
University of Barcelona; IDIBAPS, CIBERSAM, Spain

Carla Torrent

Senior Researcher, Bipolar Disorders Program,
Clinical Institute of Neuroscience,
Hospital Clinic of Barcelona;
Investigator, CIBERSAM, Spain

Anabel Martínez-Arán

Clinical Psychologist, Bipolar Disorders Program, Clinical Institute of Neuroscience,
Hospital Clinic of Barcelona; IDIBAPS, CIBERSAM, Spain

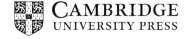

CAMBRIDGE
UNIVERSITY PRESS

CAMBRIDGE
UNIVERSITY PRESS

University Printing House, Cambridge CB2 8BS, United Kingdom

Cambridge University Press is part of the University of Cambridge.

It furthers the University's mission by disseminating knowledge in the pursuit of
education, learning and research at the highest international levels of excellence.

www.cambridge.org
Information on this title: www.cambridge.org/9781107663329

First published 2014

Printed in the United Kingdom by Clays, St Ives plc

A catalog record for this publication is available from the British Library

Library of Congress Cataloging in Publication data
Vieta, Eduard, 1963– author.
Functional remediation for bipolar disorder / Eduard Vieta, Carla Torrent, Anabel Martínez–Arán.
p. ; cm.
Includes bibliographical references and index.
ISBN 978-1-107-66332-9 (Pbk.)
I. Torrent, Carla, author. II. Martínez-Arán, Anabel, author. III. Title.
[DNLM: 1. Bipolar Disorder–rehabilitation. 2. Bipolar Disorder–psychology. 3. Cognition
Disorders–rehabilitation. 4. Cognitive Therapy–methods. WM 207]
RC516
616.89′5–dc23 2014009758

ISBN 978-1-107-66332-9 Paperback

Additional resources for this publication at www.cambridge.org/9781107663329

....

Contents

Collaborators in the creation of the functional remediation program

Brisa Solé

C. Mar Bonnín

Esther Jiménez

Imma Torres

Preface

In the 1990s, the concept that manic-depressive illness was merely a cycling condition with a virtual absence of any cognitive impairment was challenged, and since then a huge body of scientific evidence has shown that neurocognitive deficits can be detected not only during acute episodes but beyond. Many, though not all, patients with bipolar disorder have difficulties in paying attention, remembering, concentrating, learning, planning, setting priorities, and adjusting to a competitive environment. Most patients, despite being in clinical remission, report feeling vulnerable to stress and having occupational difficulties. In our clinical practice, where most of our research questions come from, we have been faced with complaints from our patients concerning their functional capacities, which have little correlation with their clinical situation. There was a clear mismatch between our perception (my job is done, the patient is well) and our patients' perception (how can I be well if I am unable to hold down a job?).

In the Bipolar Disorders Program at Barcelona we have been involved in the clinical development of most, if not all, of the currently available compounds for the treatment of bipolar disorder, seeking better treatment options for patients. We also pioneered the implementation of evidence-based psychoeducation aimed at improving awareness, treatment adherence, and patient empowerment. Those pharmacological and psychological interventions that proved useful were implemented in our clinical care program, and we could see many of the benefits that came across from those, but we remained helpless in the face of the occupational and social challenges that our patients were still reporting, and which appeared unrelated to the illness. Now we know that cognitive dysfunction is a core feature of bipolar disorder, and that, along with subclinical depressive symptoms, it is a major driver of functional impairment.

This manual represents a scientific effort to build an intervention aimed at solving the functional problems of patients with bipolar disorder. We developed this particular intervention on the basis of the cognitive deficits that we identified in several studies from a number of research groups over the world, and from our own experience with patients. The structure of the program, based on group intervention, is inspired by our psychoeducation package, which has been extremely successful and is now a crucial ingredient in the treatment of patients with bipolar illness in all international treatment guidelines. We tried to avoid "another cognitive remediation" proposal, like the many that are available for patients with schizophrenia, from which we learned that the main problem is to transfer the new neurocognitive skills to daily life. For this reason, we developed particular exercises that had a strong ecological component, with a lot of homework and practical applications. That is the foundation of *functional remediation*, as opposed to *cognitive remediation*. Ours is, indeed, a neurobehavioral approach.

These would be empty words if functional remediation had not been tested in the context of a randomized, blinded clinical trial, which is the highest standard to test any treatment. The trial (code NCT 01370668) was a multicenter study that required the training of dozens of psychologists for over a year, and tested the efficacy of functional remediation against psychoeducation and against treatment as usual, which mostly meant psychopharmacological treatment alone. The three groups received medication but different psychosocial packages, or none. The results, published in the *American Journal of Psychiatry*, showed that functional remediation made patients function better, especially in the interpersonal and occupational domains, than those who received medication only. Psychoeducation, an intervention aimed at helping patients to remain well and prevent relapse, but not specifically designed to improve their psychosocial adjustment, was neither superior to treatment as usual nor inferior to functional remediation, meaning that it had some weak effects on functioning. These findings have led us to add functional remediation therapy to the traditional "medication plus psychoeducation" approach that we provide in our specialized clinic.

This manual is divided into four chapters. The first summarizes current knowledge on cognition and functioning in bipolar disorder and provides the background for the intervention. Chapter 2 explains the potential of cognitive remediation in psychiatric disorders and the results of previous studies, mostly in the field of schizophrenia, while Chapter 3 focuses specifically on bipolar disorder and the results of the validation study. Chapter 4 explains the different modules and sessions of functional remediation, with specific guidance on how to deliver the therapy. Every session is organized according to objectives, procedures, and homework, and finally some materials are given to the patient for further learning and practice. The book also includes two appendices, giving details of the Functioning Assessment Short Test (FAST) with which functional status and progress can be tracked, and the neuropsychological battery that we use.

The tools for functional remediation are available online at www.cambridge.org/9781107663329. Those tools include PowerPoint slides for use in the group sessions, and reading materials. The intervention has been designed to be delivered in group format, but it can be used as individual therapy, with minor modifications.

We hope that this manual and the associated online tools will help healthcare professionals to be more aware of the neurocognitive and real-life problems of patients with bipolar disorder, and to try to ameliorate those problems through evidence-based functional remediation techniques. This new approach, which is at the cutting edge of psychotherapy innovation, can actually have a significant impact on patients' lives and the costs to society. The material covered in this manual is by no means intended as a theoretical textbook of neuropsychology; it is a pragmatic tool aiming to provide a foundation that can be tailored to individual requirements.

Acknowledgments

We would like to thank all those who have participated in reviewing the material for the functional remediation program and the remediation groups, including María Reinares, Clara Mercadé, and Sara Soria. The functional remediation program was made possible by the work of many people. We would like to thank all the team of the Bipolar Disorder Unit of the Hospital Clínic de Barcelona for their dedication to this project to evaluate the efficacy of functional remediation, and particularly Francesc Colom, Isabella Pacchiarotti, Jose Sánchez-Moreno, Adriane Rosa, Antoni Benabarre, Jose Manuel Goikolea, Marc Valentí, Iria Grande, Diego Hidalgo, and Juan Undurraga. This project was carried out with the collaboration of many colleagues from other centers belonging to CIBER de Salud Mental en España (Gregorio Marañón University General Hospital and Health Research Institute [IISGM]; FIDMAG Research Foundation Germanes Hospitalàries, Barcelona; Álava University Hospital, University of the Basque Country, Kronikgune, Vitoria; Department of Psychiatry, University Hospital of Bellvitge, Bellvitge Biomedical Research Institute [IDIBELL], Barcelona; Department of Medicine, University of Valencia, CIBERSAM, Valencia; Department of Psychiatry, Autonomous University of Madrid, Research Institute of the Hospital de la Princesa, Madrid; Department of Psychiatry, University of Oviedo; Department of Psychiatry, Ramon y Cajal Hospital, Alcalá University, IRYCIS, Madrid). We also want to thank Donna Pringle for the translation of the manual from Spanish to English. Finally, we would like to thank our patients and their relatives for their motivation, support, and participation in the groups. They are the heart of the program, impelling us to improve it and search for new therapeutic alternatives which will improve their functioning and quality of life.

Chapter 1

Cognition and functioning in bipolar disorder

Introduction

Over the last two decades it has been demonstrated that bipolar patients present both cognitive dysfunctions and difficulties in psychosocial functioning beyond the episodes of the disease, even during periods of mood stability (Martínez-Arán et al., 2000; Goetz et al., 2007; Sánchez-Moreno et al., 2009b). Difficulties in psychosocial functioning present especially as difficulties in adequate occupational performance and social integration, and occur not only in bipolar subtype I but also in subtype II of the disease (Ruggero et al., 2007). In a study carried out by the National Institute of Mental Health (NIMH) in the United States in the 1970s, fewer than half of the patients admitted for bipolar disorder returned to work after discharge. At two years, one-third of the patients demonstrated difficulties in work performance, and at five years even the patients who had been compensated in the previous two years presented alterations in social functioning. Along the same lines, one study analyzing the number of work days lost per year due to physical and mental diseases reported bipolar disorder to be one of the most disabling conditions, together with neurological disorders and posttraumatic stress disorder (Gitlin et al., 1995). In another European study including almost 3500 patients, psychiatrists were asked about the occupational situation of the patients one year prior to a manic episode (Goetz et al., 2007). The results indicated that 28–68% of the patients presented some degree of occupational problems, 21% of whom were totally unable to work.

Neurocognitive functions

Over the last few years there has been growing interest in the study of cognitive function in bipolar disorder. This interest has been translated into an increase in the number of publications specifically related to the cognitive performance of these patients during periods of euthymia, as well as studies of first-degree relatives of bipolar patients sharing the same genetic profile but not affected by the disease, and bipolar children and adolescents. Nonetheless, the number of studies remains low in comparison with other psychiatric diseases such as schizophrenia (Balanza-Martinez et al., 2005). It has recently become clear that there is a need to combine research efforts, integrating neuroimaging, neuropsychology, and genetic findings, in order to respond to complex questions related to vulnerability markers for bipolar disorder.

The importance of evaluating cognitive function in these patients is due to the impact that cognitive deficits may have on general functioning. For a long time it has often been considered that worse socio-occupational functioning may be the result of affective clinical or subclinical symptoms, while the effect of cognitive dysfunctions has been underestimated.

There is evidence that different cognitive areas are altered during the acute phases of the disease, especially related to tasks involving attention, memory, executive functions, and psychomotor speed, while the general intellectual level of the patients usually remains preserved, although slight changes may be observed based on the mood state of the patient. The different findings are, on occasions, contradictory, since bipolar and unipolar depression are not always differentiated. In addition, very few studies have been performed in manic patients, because of the difficulty in evaluating these patients in this state. Neurocognition studies in bipolar disorder have different limitations, and more studies are necessary in this area to help resolve many of the functioning problems of these patients.

Below we present a short review regarding which areas or cognitive domains may be altered and which are preserved during the remission periods of the disease, with special emphasis on the deficits that persist and are free of the influence of acute symptomatology.

Attention

Attention constitutes the basis for all the cognitive processes, since its alteration implies difficulties in psychomotor functions, learning, and memory as well as in executive functions.

With regard to *sustained attention* there is a certain consensus with respect to its alteration in acute bipolar patients. Based on stricter criteria for euthymia, studies over the past decade have observed persistent deficits in tasks of sustained attention in euthymic bipolar patients (Clark *et al.*, 2002), suggesting that this type of dysfunction may be a marker of disease trait. However, there is controversy as to whether it could be strictly considered as a cognitive endophenotype, taking into account the contradictory results found in first-degree relatives of bipolar patients not affected by the disease, using a range of measures related to the Continuous Performance Test (CPT) as a reference to assess sustained attention (Arts *et al.*, 2008; Bora *et al.*, 2009). On the other hand, it seems clear that the deficit in sustained attention is present at disease onset, as has been detected in a sample of patients who had recently recuperated from a first manic episode (Torres *et al.*, 2007), as well as in a study including a sample of bipolar patients with a disease duration of less than five years and with a maximum of two affective episodes (Kolur *et al.*, 2006). Since there is practically no information on the cognitive performance of patients prior to manifestation of the disease, attention deficits supposedly become more evident over time, although they may be present at the onset of the disease.

With regard to *selective attention,* a deficit has been observed in the active periods of the disease. In some studies improvement has been described in measures of attention after the remission of clinical symptoms, suggesting that the difficulty in focusing attention may be a sensitive indicator of clinical status. Nonetheless, other studies suggest that a deficit in selective attention may be maintained in depressed patients, despite a clear clinical improvement six months after hospital discharge. In other studies undertaken in euthymic bipolar patients a deficit in selective attention was not reported. The deficits found in other measures with an attention component, such as the Trail Making Test (TMT), were attributed to alterations in working memory. More recent investigations have described attentional dysfunctions in patients with schizophrenia, and in bipolar patients as well as their first-degree relatives compared with healthy controls on performing the Stroop Color and Word Test (SCWT). In recent years a number of studies have detected a worse performance in the measurement of interference in the Stroop test in acute patients and in those in remission, which seems to be maintained in the long term (Kronhaus *et al.*, 2006), even demonstrating a similar grade of involvement to that of schizophrenic patients (Balanza-Martinez *et al.*, 2005). Indeed, an altered inhibitory response has been proposed as the most evident endophenotype candidate in bipolar disorder (Bora *et al.*, 2009). These findings may be linked with others more recently published that demonstrate alterations in the patterns of cerebral activation in euthymic bipolar patients compared with healthy controls using functional magnetic resonance (fMR) during the Stroop test, showing reduced ventromedial prefrontal cortex activity (Kronhaus *et al.*, 2006).

Working memory

Working memory is a storage system with limited capacity that allows manipulation of information, facilitating the performance of several cognitive tasks simultaneously. Different authors consider working memory as the basic cognitive deficit in schizophrenia. Nevertheless, investigations increasingly indicate that bipolar patients also present difficulties in tasks requiring verbal working memory (e.g., the Digit Span WAIS) as well as in other visual or spatial tests of working memory in both the acute phases of the disease and in euthymia. According to a study by Glahn and collaborators (2006) comparing schizophrenic, schizoaffective, and bipolar psychotic and non-psychotic patients, the spatial working memory distinguishes patients with psychotic symptomatology from non-psychotic patients.

Memory

The tests most frequently used for the assessment of verbal memory in bipolar disorder are related to word lists or remembering stories.

In general, deficits of learning and memory have been associated both with the acute phase of the disease and with periods of euthymia (Martínez-Arán et al., 2004b; Robinson and Ferrier, 2006). Mnemonic dysfunctions may be sensitive to subtle subsyndromic fluctuations, particularly of the depressive type, which is why some studies have proposed that these difficulties are not detectable once the effect of the subclinical symptomatology has been controlled for. Nonetheless, recent studies in which the effect of the subsyndromic affective symptomatology has been controlled for have reported the presence of alterations in verbal memory as possible markers of trait or cognitive endophenotypes. The consensus on alterations in verbal memory in euthymic patients is increasingly greater (Glahn et al., 2004; Robinson and Ferrier, 2006; Balanza-Martinez et al., 2008; Bora et al., 2009). One study observed that depressed and hypomanic bipolar patients differ in respect of the nature of the verbal dysfunctions: whereas depressed patients present a greater difficulty in recognition tasks, hypomanic patients present more difficulties in long-term memory (Malhi et al., 2007).

An investigative team in Cincinnati reported that both euthymic and manic patients demonstrate difficulties in remembering information in learning tests based on word lists, such as the California Verbal Learning Test (CVLT) (Fleck et al., 2003); although only manic patients present difficulties in the recognition task, thereby making difficulties in information encoding more marked in these patients, euthymic bipolar patients probably present more difficulties in the retrieval of information. Bipolar patients most likely present difficulties in the organization of verbal information during the encoding process, that is, they have problems in using semantic encoding strategies. In a recent meta-analysis, moderate to large effect sizes were found in verbal memory, especially in verbal learning and in both immediate and delayed free memory (Torres et al., 2007). In a comparison of the neuropsychological performance of schizophrenic and bipolar patients with respect to verbal memory, the bipolar patients showed fewer dysfunctions than the schizophrenic patients (Daban et al., 2006c).

On the other hand, as reflected in the International Society for Bipolar Disorders–Battery for Assessment of Neurocognition (ISBD-BANC), some tests have shown greater sensitivity in detecting verbal memory dysfunctions in these patients, such as the CVLT compared with other types of tools. One of the main reasons for finding more deficits with the CVLT is that this test incorporates the use of strategies involving an executive component, which means that the subjects can semantically organize the information to better remember it. This overlapping of verbal memory and executive functions is more marked with this test than with other verbal memory tasks such as the Auditory Verbal Learning Test (AVLT) or the Rey Auditory Verbal Learning Test (RAVLT).

With regard to visual memory, in some patients this function is impaired in the acute phases of the disease, particularly in those with a previous history of psychosis or in bipolar patients evaluated during the first episode with psychotic symptoms, according to the subscale of visual memory of the Wechsler Memory Scale (WMS) or similar tasks (Albus et al., 1996). Among the scarce studies carried out in bipolar children and adolescents, impairments have been described in measures of visual–spatial memory that cannot be explained by the presence of affective symptomatology or comorbidity with attention-deficit hyperactivity disorder (ADHD). Again, the findings are more discrepant when referring to bipolar patients in remission. Although some studies have observed persistent deficits in euthymic patients with the WMS and the Delayed Matching to Sample Task (DMST), it seems that most of the studies performed did not find cognitive dysfunctions in the area of visual memory; and when reported in euthymic patients, the difficulties disappear after controlling for the effect of the subdepressive symptomatology.

One of the most consistent findings is the dissociation between explicit or declarative and implicit or procedural memory. While the first is impaired in bipolar disorder, procedural memory is preserved, similar to what occurs in unipolar depression.

Some investigations have shown that relatives not affected by the disease also seem to present difficulties in learning and verbal memory, albeit to a lesser degree. These results therefore support the contention that mnemonic dysfunctions in this area constitute a trait marker of the disease. The presence of subtle deficits indicates that cognitive deficits may represent a factor of vulnerability in the development of bipolar disorder, since they may be present at the onset of the disease but may worsen with the illness course, as will be shown later.

Executive functions

Again, there is discrepancy among the different authors with respect to the performance of bipolar patients in tasks related to executive functions. Executive dysfunction has also been observed in euthymic bipolar patients, especially in the number of persistent errors which they make in tasks such as the Wisconsin Card Sorting Test (WCST). In addition, euthymic bipolar patients correctly complete fewer categories in this same test, especially in the case of comorbid alcohol dependence (van Gorp et al., 1998). In relation to other frontal function tests such as the verbal fluency tasks, a deficit is generally observed in the depressive state, mainly with reference to phonetic fluency, although there is usually no deficit during the manias, with discordance regarding findings in patients in remission. In general, the difficulties in verbal fluency usually improve and even normalize during periods of euthymia.

Recent meta-analyses (Torres et al., 2007; Arts et al., 2008; Bora et al., 2009) have shown that bipolar patients present significantly lower results in executive function tests than healthy subjects. The deficits observed were not due to differences related to premorbid intelligence quotient (IQ) or years of education. The executive dysfunctions, especially in tasks requiring inhibitory control, constitute a very important trait marker of bipolar disorder, independently of the severity of the disorder and the medication. Deficits in different executive functions are present from the onset of the disease (Torres et al., 2010), and even the recurrence of manic episodes may have a long-term neurocognitive impact on executive function (López-Jaramillo et al., 2010a). On the other hand, Frangou and colleagues (2005) also found that alterations in executive function represent a trait marker for bipolar disorder, but that the factors related to these impairments are treatment with antipsychotic drugs, disease chronicity, and the level of symptomatology presented.

Therefore, the executive dysfunctions seem to persist at least in a subgroup of patients independently of the clinical state (Martínez-Arán et al., 2004a; Balanza-Martinez et al., 2005; Robinson and Ferrier, 2006; López-Jaramillo et al., 2010a). Some investigators have conceptualized the deficit in "frontal" function tasks as an alteration in the executive control of working memory. Executive alterations reflect the presence of underlying structural or functional neuroanatomical dysfunctions in the prefrontal cortex. Differences have been described in the general cortical or prefrontal volume, in particular, between patients and healthy subjects. According to the results of most of the studies published, alterations may be found in the dorsolateral anterior cingulate prefrontal cortex.

Psychomotor performance

Motor performance has been scarcely studied in bipolar disorder. Greater psychomotor slowing has been described in depressive bipolar than in unipolar patients. In studies comparing euthymic bipolar patients with healthy controls, the deficit reportedly persisted during euthymia even after controlling for the residual depressive symptoms using tests such as the TMT-A or the Digit Symbol Substitution Test (DSST). A deficit has been observed in coordination and motor sequencing. Nonetheless, other authors have not reported differences in performance between euthymic patients and controls. Some studies have described psychomotor speed deficits both in bipolar patients and in healthy first-degree relatives. Thus, together with the executive functions, psychomotor functioning is considered as a cognitive phenotype of bipolar disorder (Antila *et al.*, 2007). Study of motor speed, as well as information processing speed, needs greater attention, since it is probably affected in these patients. Future investigations are required to shed light on this aspect.

Other cognitive functions

Although there is a lack of studies in this area to date, bipolar patients present impairments in the processing of information with emotional content; for example, with regard to recognition of facial expressions, even euthymic patients demonstrate difficulty, and it is thereby considered a stable deficit. One recent study reported that bipolar patients show a biased response, mainly towards information of negative content (Gopin *et al.*, 2011). This altered pattern of cognitive–social skills suggests a dysfunction of the neuronal circuits that mediate the emotional, social, and linguistic–pragmatic processes (appropriate social use of verbal and non-verbal language).

Despite the greater interest that has arisen concerning social cognition in bipolar disorder, a great deal remains to be investigated. Impairments have been detected in the theory of mind in euthymic bipolar patients, although it has been proposed that the deficits presented may be mediated, in part, by attention deficits or executive dysfunction. On the other hand, the evidence available seems to indicate that patients in acute phases of the disease present difficulties in decision making. Likewise, some studies have reported that patients in remission may also present difficulties of this type, although there are some discrepancies. There seems to be a relation between impairment in decision making and the history of suicide attempt, probably as a risk factor of vulnerability. Neuroimaging studies have demonstrated the involvement of the ventro-medial prefrontal cortex as well as the amygdala in decision making. The processing of emotional–social information is more linked to the orbitofrontal cortex, limbic system, and, especially, the amygdala, in addition to the anterior cingulate. It is also possible that these measures are related more to psychosocial functioning, and therefore to the problems that patients may present in the social and occupational areas.

One field that has begun to be investigated in the last few years, and in which much remains to be done, is the implication of the default mode network. This network is a group of cerebral regions that collaborate among themselves and are very active during rest but deactivate for performing a cognitive task. The default mode network is located in the medial parts of the hemispheres, specifically in the medial prefrontal cortex and the posterior cingulate cortex, among other zones. The few studies that have been carried out suggest a dysfunction in the default mode network in bipolar disorder similar to what has been detected in other psychiatric disorders such as schizophrenia or autism. People with psychosis present problems at the time of disconnecting this network when it is necessary to respond to an external stimulus or concentrate on a cognitive task. Defects in activation are also detected. These may turn out to be key findings in understanding mental diseases and in finding their cerebral bases (Pomarol-Clotet *et al.*, 2012).

Table 1.1 shows the cognitive domains most affected in bipolar disorder, the anatomical structures involved, and the neuropsychological tests used.

Factors associated with cognitive dysfunctions

Different factors are related to the clinical, pharmacological, and prognostic variables which may be directly or indirectly related to cognitive functioning in patients with bipolar disorder (Table 1.2).

Table 1.1 Cognitive domains affected in bipolar disorder, anatomical structures involved, and neuropsychological tests used

Neurocognitive domain	Neuroanatomical structure	Test
Attention		CPT, TMT-A, WAIS-III Digit Span Forward
Sustained attention	Orbitofrontal lateral, dorsolateral prefrontal cortex, basal ganglia	CPT
Divided attention	Anterior cingulate, dorsolateral prefrontal cortex	TMT
Inhibition/decision making	Orbitofrontal cortex, anterior cingulate	Stroop, GO-NoGo, Iowa Gambling Test
Spatial/verbal working memory	Superior parietal lobe, dorsolateral prefrontal cortex	WAIS-III Digit Spatial Span, WMS-III Letter-Number sequencing, N-back
Verbal fluency	Prefrontal cortex	FAS (COWAT), Animal Naming
Motor speed/skill	Subcortical ganglia, basal ganglia	TMT-A, TMT-B
Memory (encoding, storage, retrieval, recall)	Hippocampus, prefrontal cortex, ventromedial prefrontal cortex, temporoparietal junction	CVLT, CVLT-II, WMS-III Logical Memory
Executive function		
Logical reasoning	Left frontal cortex, temporal cortex	WCST
Cognitive control	Ventrolateral and dorsolateral prefrontal cortex, anterior cingulate	Stroop
Set shifting	Cerebellum, left dorsolateral prefrontal cortex, basal ganglia	TMT-B, WCST, Stroop

Table 1.2 Principal factors associated with cognitive dysfunctions in bipolar disorder

- Subclinical symptoms
- Disease duration
- Number of episodes (especially manic)
- Psychotic symptoms
- Hormonal factors
- Comorbidity (substance intake, anxiety)
- Medication
- Stress
- Sleep disorders
- Other factors (diagnostic subtype, substance abuse and dependence . . .)

Subclinical symptoms

Most bipolar patients are symptomatic most of the time, despite following pharmacological treatment. The presence of subsyndromic symptomatology may influence the general level of functioning. The subsyndromic symptomatology probably has a specific weight in cognitive functioning in addition to a negative influence on psychosocial functioning. However, the direction of causality is not very clear, since patients with the greatest number of psychosocial difficulties also possibly develop more depressive symptomatology. In any case, bipolar patients should be evaluated when in clinical remission to avoid the confounding effect of the affective symptoms.

Disease duration

The years of disease evolution also seem to have a relevant role in cognitive functioning in these patients, despite the discrepancies between the different studies. Chronicity, understood as duration of the disease, has been associated with greater memory deficits, although mnemonic dysfunction may also be a predictor of chronicity. Despite the scarce longitudinal studies in this field, there are progressively more contributions on the relevance of chronicity in cognitive function in bipolar disorder. In fact, a systematic review reported that of 11 studies which had analyzed the impact of chronicity on cognitive functioning, approximately half found a relation between disease duration and different cognitive variables related to psychomotor speed, visual–spatial memory, and, in particular, verbal memory (Robinson and Ferrier, 2006).

Number of episodes

The number of relapses presented by a bipolar patient may also have a negative influence on cognitive function. The impact, such as negative consequences on functioning and quality of life, that each episode has on cognition is by no means benign, and thus, for this and other reasons, it is important to prevent relapse. Different authors have found correlations between neuropsychological deficits and a greater number of episodes or a worse disease evolution (Robinson and Ferrier, 2006). Manic episodes seem to be associated with cognitive deficits, and they may have a neurotoxic effect mainly on the hippocampus and prefrontal cortex, reducing the number of glucocorticoid receptors and leading to greater cognitive dysfunction (Ferrier and Thompson, 2002). Several studies have observed that the greater the number of manic phases, the worse the performance in measures of verbal memory and executive functions as well as in measures of attention. Nonetheless, cognitive deficits may be present from the onset of the illness, as has been observed in a sample of patients in remission following the first manic episode. The findings compared to depressive phases are not as consistent, but 60% of the studies analyzing the relationship between depressive episodes and neuropsychological variables also found negative correlations (Robinson and Ferrier, 2006). The concept of "allostatic load" may help to explain the negative effects that repeated episodes produce, increasing and involving alterations at a molecular level that are translated into an impact on neurocognition.

Psychotic symptoms

The presence of psychotic symptoms, or, more specifically, a previous history of psychotic symptomatology, may be associated with worse cognitive function in bipolar patients (Martínez-Arán *et al.*, 2004a, 2008; Daban *et al.*, 2006a). Nonetheless, contrary to this hypothesis, some findings associate the cognitive deficit in schizophrenia with negative syndromes and disorganization. Moreover, the cognitive deficit in schizophrenia is characterized by its stability, independently of the psychotic symptoms. Studies have been performed in patients with first episodes with and without psychotic symptoms, and it has been observed that those presenting psychotic symptoms, independently of the diagnosis (unipolar or bipolar disorders or schizophrenia), achieved a worse performance than patients without psychotic symptoms. Along the same lines, the findings of other studies indicate that psychotic symptomatology has a negative influence on performance in a large proportion of the neuropsychological tests, especially those related to executive functions (Bora *et al.*, 2007; Glahn *et al.*, 2007) and verbal memory (Martínez-Arán *et al.*, 2007). A recent meta-analysis also pointed in the same direction, although the effect of the psychotic symptoms did not, by itself, explain the cognitive dysfunction in bipolar patients (Bora *et al.*, 2010).

Hormonal factors

Hypercortisolemia may be present during manic and depressive phases of bipolar disorder. Some studies have suggested that elevated cortisol levels may produce lesions in the hippocampus, even after remission of the acute episode, which may lead to dysfunctions, especially in declarative memory. Atrophy and loss of hippocampal neurons may be induced by stress.

The potential neurotoxic effects of hypercortisolemia could explain, in part, that the course of the disease may become complicated with each episode and that manic episodes may be closely related to cognitive deficits. On the other hand, one of the mechanisms contributing to the negative impact of stress is the regulation of neurotrophic factors such as BDNF (brain-derived neurotrophic factor), which is necessary for neuron survival and function. Sustained reduction of this factor contributes to the neurotoxic effect of stress on the brain. Both acute and chronic stress influences a reduction in cerebral neuroplasticity. In addition, a reduction in BDNF has been associated with poorer performance of memory tests and executive functions (Kapczinski *et al.*, 2008a).

Patients medicated with lithium and presenting subclinical hypothyroidism showed worse performance in verbal learning and memory tests compared with patients without thyroid alterations (Tremont and Stern, 1997, 2000). Similar results have been obtained in other studies, observing that the side effects improve in patients treated with thyroxine and that the performance of neuropsychological tasks are more correlated with the serum levels of thyrotrophin than with those of lithium.

Medication

The effect of pharmacological treatment is difficult to assess in bipolar patients, since they usually follow combined treatments at variable doses.

The negative effects of lithium on cognition seem to be lesser and of little importance, emphasizing the current study on the neuroprotective effects of lithium. In a recent study, no neuropsychological differences were observed when comparing patients treated with lithium monotherapy with patients without pharmacological treatment, thereby indicating that the neurocognitive deficits are not explained by the treatment (López-Jaramillo *et al.*, 2010b). Likewise, in a longitudinal study over a six-year period, no differences were found between the patients receiving and not receiving lithium, demonstrating stable neuropsychological performance (Engelsmann *et al.*, 1988).

With respect to anticonvulsants, there is little evidence of cognitive deficits, although a deficit in concentration has been described with valproate or carbamazepine. Among the new antiepileptics, lamotrigine and gabapentin seem to demonstrate a better cognitive profile in epileptic patients, and some preliminary data available on bipolar patients favor lamotrigine with respect to cognitive performance compared with conventional antiepileptics (Daban *et al.*, 2006b).

In relation to antipsychotics, the use of conventional antipsychotics may have a negative effect on short-term motor function, although a beneficial effect may be produced in the long-term surveillance and visual processing of information. Most authors agree that antipsychotics do not improve cognitive function, but neither do they worsen it, and that even the cognitive side effects are related more to the use of anticholinergic medication than to antipsychotics. However, their effect in bipolar patients requires further study, since most research has been undertaken in schizophrenic patients. The incorporation of new antipsychotics will probably help to improve these cognitive dysfunctions, although the cognitive function will most likely not normalize in these patients.

With respect to antidepressants there is little clear evidence showing a worsening in cognitive function, and, in general, they have a positive cognitive profile, except for those in which the anticholinergic effects are greater.

Finally, benzodiazepines, which are normally used to treat insomnia and anxiety in these patients, may produce memory, attention, and motor speed dysfunctions, if the administration is prolonged.

Nonetheless, the cognitive dysfunctions observed in bipolar patients do not seem to be due only to the medication, and thus it cannot be stated that they are exclusively a pharmacologic by-product. Cognitive deficits are largely related to the disease itself, as demonstrated in the scarce studies performed in non-medicated patients and in investigations with first-degree relatives. The truth is that most of the data referring to the effects of the medication on cognition have been achieved in samples including schizophrenic or epileptic patients and, in most cases, in healthy volunteers, but little is known about how it affects bipolar patients from a neurocognitive point of view. Although the cognitive deficit in bipolar disorder does not seem to be a primary effect of treatment, it cannot be ruled out that some treatments have a certain impact on cognitive functions, especially in the case of high doses or combined treatments.

Other factors

Substance abuse and dependence is associated with a worse course of the disease and may affect cognitive function. Comorbid alcohol dependence has been associated with worse performance on measures of executive function and verbal memory, although the deficits are generally related more to the bipolar disorder itself than to the premorbid disorder of alcohol abuse or dependence (Sánchez-Moreno et al., 2009a).

Other factors which may be related to greater cognitive dysfunction are rapid cycling, although this relationship has been little studied, the number of hospitalizations indirectly associated with the severity of the course of the disease, the family history of affective or psychotic disorders, and sleep alterations, which may also influence memory function.

The diagnostic subtype is also interesting to study, given the paucity of data on this aspect; in general, studies of cognitive deficits have been undertaken either in bipolar I patients or in heterogeneous patients, including both bipolar I and II. The scientific literature suggests that bipolar II patients also present cognitive deficits, although perhaps of a lesser grade than type I patients in some cognitive domains (Torrent et al., 2006; Sole et al., 2012). There is a growing interest in the need to differentiate subgroups at a neuropsychological level. On comparing the schizoaffective disorder versus bipolar patients without psychotic symptoms and healthy controls, worse cognitive function was observed in the schizoaffective patients (Torrent et al., 2007). Therefore, cognitive dysfunctions are observed along the whole bipolar spectrum, supporting the hypothesis of a continuum among the affective disorders and the schizophrenic spectrum.

Neurodevelopment or neuroprogression?

There are many doubts as to whether cognitive deficits are present prior to the onset of the disease, which would favor the hypothesis of alterations in neurodevelopment. On the other hand, it may be the impact of the disease itself that negatively influences cognition, which would support the hypothesis of cognitive impairment or a neurodegenerative process. Nonetheless, the two processes may possibly be compatible. From a neuropsychological point of view, follow-up studies of more than one year in these patients are scarce. It seems that the deficits are maintained, but it is complicated to establish whether this impairment is stable or progressive.

Some subtle neurocognitive deficits are probably present prior to the onset of the disease, although few studies have been carried out in populations at high risk of having bipolar disorder. Nonetheless, according to the findings available at present, the hypothesis of neurodevelopment seems to be the more plausible for schizophrenia than for bipolar disorder. In one of the studies undertaken in Dunedin (New Zealand), the subjects later diagnosed with bipolar disorder showed higher premorbid intellectual function than schizophrenic subjects, with a similar or even higher function than healthy controls (Cannon et al., 2002). Other studies carried out in Sweden and Israel showed similar findings (Reichenberg et al., 2002; Zammit et al., 2004). However, recent investigations performed in the University of Valencia and in the Institute of Neurosciences in the Miguel Hernández University in Alicante, Spain, have suggested the possibility that at least a small percentage of bipolar patients may present alterations linked to neurodevelopment. These contributions are of extraordinary interest, since they suggest that a subgroup of bipolar patents and schizophrenic patients present mutations in genes implicated in neuronal migration, and these anomalies may even predict the presence of executive dysfunctions in these patients (Tabares-Seisdedos et al., 2006).

In recent years, in the search for candidate endophenotypes, there has been increasing interest in the possibility that cognitive dysfunctions are also present in first-degree relatives of bipolar patients. If the neuropsychological deficits found in the patients were a phenotypic expression of genetic vulnerability to bipolar disorder, healthy subjects with a genetic predisposition for this disease would be expected to manifest the same deficits. Among the studies carried out in adults with a genetic risk of having bipolar disorder, most demonstrated mild impairments in different components of executive functions (planning, inhibition, or cognitive flexibility) and verbal memory (Thompson et al., 2005). Nonetheless, a recent investigation based on a multigenerational study with a wide sample of families suggested genetically correlated and significantly heritable measures related to processing speed, working memory, and declarative memory (facial) as potential endophenotypes (Glahn et al., 2010). Likewise, studies performed in twins of bipolar patients without the disease have shown a deficit in working memory and in delayed memory of verbal information. At the same time, worse academic performance has been observed in the children of bipolar patients, suggesting a certain grade of cognitive involvement in children in the absence of clinical symptoms but with a high risk of developing the disease. In another study, discordance was observed between verbal and manipulative IQ, with better performance in the former. These arguments imply the possibility that there are cognitive endophenotypes that are trait markers of the disease, and therefore possible biological markers in the psychopathology of bipolar disorder.

We are still in the initial stages, and it is too early to draw conclusions. Future studies will probably provide greater clarity as to whether the deficit is present prior to the onset of bipolar disorder, is a consequence of the disease itself, or is a product of the combination of the two. According to some authors, memory impairments depend more on the clinical state at an early age, and with time convert into a trait due to the neurotoxicity associated with multiple episodes which affect the functioning of the prefrontal and medial temporal cortex. This neurotoxic model would imply that through pathological levels of cortisol, multiple relapses lead to neurostructural changes, which may be accompanied by cognitive dysfunctions that persist after clinical remission. The patient recovers from the episode, but the anatomical alterations undergo a slow recovery or may even be irreversible. At present, however, this interpretation remains speculative, and further, more rigorous, investigations are required to confirm the hypothesis.

With regard to the early phases, deficits in sustained attention, learning and memory, spatial reasoning, and in some executive functions have been described in euthymic patients following the first episode of mania. In one of these studies the cognitive deficit was associated more with the fact of having presented psychotic symptoms during the episode than with the diagnosis. In another study with a two-year follow-up after the first affective episode, bipolar patients presented very few cognitive dysfunctions.

The great problem in the study of the evolution of cognitive dysfunctions in bipolar disorder is that these have been studied from a cross-sectional perspective, and few longitudinal follow-ups of more than one year have been performed, although there are some, albeit very few, studies which have evaluated patients in the acute phase and in remission around one year and eight months later. None of these studies found progressive cognitive impairment. In stable patients, Balanza-Martinez and collaborators (2005) observed persistent deficits in 12 of the 13 cognitive measures compared with normal controls. Other data from a two-year follow-up study in euthymic bipolar patients treated largely with lithium monotherapy can be added to these data (Mur et al., 2008). The findings suggest persistent deficits in executive functions and processing speed, despite an average time of euthymia of three years in this sample. These results suggest that neurocognitive deficits are maintained even when the inter-episode periods are prolonged. In another longitudinal study with a mean follow-up of nine years, persistence in cognitive deficits was observed in all the domains except in the executive functions, in which a worsening was described (Torrent et al., 2012).

It is evident that more longitudinal studies are required to elucidate the evolution of cognitive dysfunctions in bipolar patients, since the data obtained to date are too scarce to conclude that the deficits worsen over time. Indeed, the most we can say is that the deficits persist in the long term. One of the most consistent findings is that the dysfunctions, especially in verbal memory

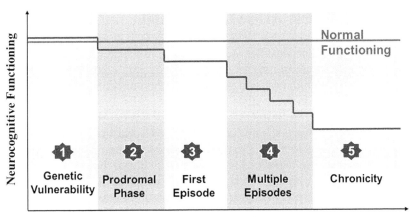

Figure 1.1 Neurocognitive evolution and disease. In the case of bipolar disorder there is genetic predisposition (1). Prior to the onset of the disease, the subject may present subtle neurocognitive deficits (2). Mnemonic alterations appear in the first episodes of the disorder (3), which convert into a cognitive trait due to the neurotoxicity produced by multiple episodes (4) over time; these latter particularly affect the prefrontal and medial temporal cortex. With time the alterations become chronic (5).

and executive functions, are probably those associated with a worse evolution, with a correlation being observed between the deficit in these cognitive domains and multiple relapses. Thus, the most chronic patients with multiple episodes have a greater probability of presenting cognitive deficits than younger patients with fewer relapses. Nonetheless, as previously mentioned, only longitudinal studies can answer whether the deficits are or are not progressive, confirming the neurodegenerative hypothesis, although in the case of bipolar disorder the concept of neuroprogression would be more appropriate than neurodegeneration (Berk *et al.*, 2007) (Figure 1.1).

Cognitive deficits and psychosocial function

Contrary to what has been believed until very recently, cognitive deficits could be more related to bad general functioning of the patient than to the symptoms of the disease itself. Although a possible negative influence of the subclinical symptoms on social and occupational adaptation of the bipolar patient has been reported, cognitive factors may have a greater predictive power and should, therefore, not be underevaluated by the clinician or confounded with residual depressive symptoms. It is important to assess if there really is a cognitive deficit, optimize the pharmacological treatment whenever possible, and search for other strategies or interventions to improve these difficulties, always with the goal of the functional recovery of the patient. The implementation of adapted neurocognitive remediation techniques is thus necessary, with the aim of reducing the cognitive deficits and thereby improving the quality of life of our patients. In any case, psychoeducational programs are of great utility in improving awareness of the disease and therapeutic compliance, and for preventing relapses, avoiding or reducing the cognitive impairment associated with the process of the disease. On the other hand, neurocognitive remediation programs are a therapeutic strategy aimed not only at improving cognitive performance but also at achieving the functional recovery of the bipolar patient. A recent multicenter randomized clinical trial demonstrated the efficacy of an intervention aimed at improving the psychosocial functioning of bipolar patients. This intervention involved training in neurocognitive techniques and strategies aimed at neurocognitive deficits, and psychoeducation concerning the deficits associated with the disorder as well as in problem solving within an ecological framework, in order to facilitate their transfer to real life (Torrent *et al.*, 2013).

Theoretical model: allostatic load

The pathophysiology of bipolar disorder is increasingly understood, although there are, for example, neurobiological questions and mechanisms linked with comorbidity, physical diseases, or cognitive involvement that remain to be elucidated. The concepts of allostasis and allostatic load may facilitate knowledge in these areas.

The concept of allostatic load was first introduced by McEwen and Stellar (1993), and was defined as the cost of chronic exposure to the fluctuation or increase of neural activity for adaptation to stress. Allostatic load implies the numerous series of modifications that the organism implements against stressors from the environment to adapt to the change, avoiding damage to the organism and its different structures at all processing levels (cells, tissues, organs, and systems).

The allostatic or adaptive systems allow response to different, not necessarily psychological, situations such as remaining awake, hunger, or doing exercise. Allostasis is the capacity to maintain stability in the face of change. Nonetheless, when the adaptive response is insufficient to achieve homeostasis, or if it is excessive, the events that should lead to a normal state stabilize in unfavorable or bad adaptive plastic changes that make up the different states of allostatic overload and its manifestations in the central nervous system and in the immune, endocrine, and cardiovascular systems.

The effects of excessive load on most of the adaptive systems of the human body are cumulative and are observed during chronic stress and aging. Bipolar disorder may be considered as a disease characterized by cumulative allostatic states in which the allostatic load increases with the increase in stressors, the involvement of the mood state, and substance intake. Each episode leads to an increase in oxidative stress, a reduction in BDNF, and an increase in inflammatory markers. This leads to a loss of neural connectivity, with cognitive impairment and with fewer resources of the individual to deal with the surrounding challenges. Thus, the paradigm of allostatic load would allow the understanding of questions related to the physiopathology of the disease such as vulnerability to stress, cognitive involvement, mortality, and the presence of comorbidities (Kapczinski *et al.*, 2008b; Vieta *et al.*, 2013) (Figure 1.2).

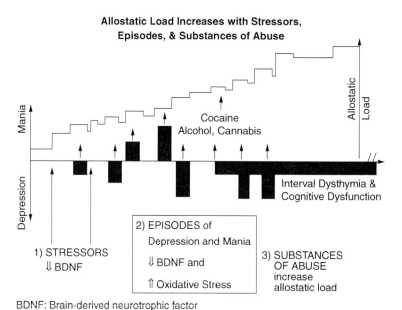

BDNF: Brain-derived neurotrophic factor

Figure 1.2 Allostatic load progressively increases with intermittent episodes as a function of cumulative stressors, mood episodes, and exposure to drugs of abuse. Increased load engenders cognitive impairment, inter-episodic subsyndromal symptoms, and increased rates of physical and psychiatric comorbidities. Initial episodes are triggered by stressors but become autonomous as the disease progresses.

The long-term consequences of the damage generated by the increase in allostatic load, the reduction in BDNF, and the stress observed during the involvement of the mood state vary, and may include telomeric shortening, an effect on neuroplasticity and cell resilience, and cognitive deficits such as difficulties in verbal memory that affect the psychosocial functioning of the patient. In turn, the systemic changes observed in bipolar patients coincide with the increase in the prevalence of chronic clinical diseases and with premature aging. In this context, allostatic load may function as a nexus between the effects of stress on brain tissue and the cellular damage resulting from the involvement of the mood state. It may be suggested that the increase in this load predisposes to the appearance of diseases such as diabetes, hypertension, and cancer.

It is necessary to perfect the diagnostic and therapeutic strategies applied to bipolar patients. The presence of a progressive increase in allostatic load may be considered in patients treated inadequately. This provides an opportunity to reassess therapeutic strategies, with the aim of contemplating the application of earlier interventions and preventive strategies maintained over time.

Chapter 2

Cognitive remediation in psychiatric disorders

Introduction

Neuropsychological remediation has made great progress in the last few years. In the beginning, the objective of remediation was to establish treatment programs for recovery of the intellectual, cognitive, emotional, behavioral, motor, executive, and social functions of the individual who had undergone neurological damage or a cerebral lesion such as cranioencephalic injuries, ictus, dementias, and brain tumors. Later, over the last two decades, there has been enormous interest in describing the neurocognitive deficits associated with mental diseases, their influence on autonomy and the quality of life of the patient, and the possible potential of pharmacological treatments and remediation to improve those deficits.

In the 1990s, the investigation of patients with schizophrenia was widely developed from previous work in patients with neurological disorders. Different studies demonstrated that neurocognitive dysfunction represents a nuclear characteristic of schizophrenia, and that it is not caused by other collateral aspects but rather is an intrinsic part of the disease, in addition to being the epicenter of many of the functional difficulties presented by patients with schizophrenia. With respect to bipolar disorder, it has been shown that bipolar patients present both cognitive dysfunctions and difficulties in psychosocial functioning beyond the episodes of the disease itself, contrary to the initial belief that patients with bipolar disorder achieve complete syndromic and functional recovery between episodes.

Cognitive remediation (CR) had been proposed as an effective treatment tool in psychiatric remediation, but a clear definition was not proposed until very recently. In 2010 the Cognitive Remediation Experts Workshop defined CR as an intervention based on behavioral training, directed at improving cognitive processes (attention, memory, executive functions, social cognition, or metacognition) with the objective of achieving permanence and generalization of this improvement (Wykes and Spaulding, 2011). In other words, CR is a psychological treatment that attempts to improve neurocognitive functioning, involves a learning process, and attempts to influence psychosocial functioning (Penadés and Gastó, 2010). Different studies have demonstrated that the presence of cognitive symptoms may impede complete functional recovery (Green et al., 2000), leading to difficulties in the development of work and school activities and in the everyday life activities of patients. Indeed, the persistence of cognitive dysfunction explains the difficulties in functioning better than the clinical symptoms per se.

The impact of CR on functioning is important, since the main reason for CR is to improve psychosocial functioning, although, surprisingly, in the case of schizophrenia, for example, this hypothesis was not investigated until the last decade. Prior to this, investigation was fundamentally focused on cognitive performance. It is therefore necessary to study and identify the specific cognitive domains related to cognitive improvement, in order to establish the appropriate objectives on which an intervention should be focused (Penadés and Gastó, 2010). CR is therefore not reduced to a specific isolated intervention on the different cognitive processes.

The appearance of training techniques in psychosocial skills marked a turning point in the field of CR for psychiatric patients, representing a first attempt to provide and teach basic life skills such as social interaction, management of the disease, autonomy, and leisure skills. However, people with cognitive deficits such as attention problems show difficulties in the acquisition of these types of skills in these programs, because of the difficulties they experience in processing and remembering the information provided in the groups, such that they are unable to maintain their attention throughout the sessions.

According to the results of a number of meta-analyses, CR programs lead to a significant, albeit moderate, change in cognitive functioning and in the maintenance of this improvement (Kurtz *et al.*, 2001; Medalia *et al.*, 2002; Pilling *et al.*, 2002; Krabbendam and Aleman, 2003; Twamley *et al.*, 2003; Bell *et al.*, 2005; McGurk *et al.*, 2007; Grynszpan *et al.*, 2011).

Cognitive remediation is not intended to replace pharmacological or psychological therapy, but rather offers a new therapeutic approach that is complementary to other interventions such as psychoeducation programs, promoting integral treatment of the disease. Nonetheless, it should also be mentioned that the currently available pharmacological treatments have a limited effect on cognition in schizophrenia, and their influence at the functioning level is even lower.

Cognitive remediation in schizophrenia

The great variety of CR programs developed for schizophrenia vary in regard to their theoretical foundations, as well as in the modalities of intervention, and there is as yet no consensus as to the essential elements of the intervention. Despite this, there are numerous similarities between the programs which probably contribute to the global benefits. The multiple programs differ in the name and method of performance: some have exercises with pencil and paper, others are computerized, with or without therapy, have a group or individual format, and have a fixed or adaptable curricular content, etc. The CR programs developed for schizophrenia have attempted to approach cognitive impairment through a great variety of methods such as instruction and practical exercises, compensatory strategies, and discussion groups. Nonetheless, the results of various meta-analyses have suggested that the differences between the specific programs are not as relevant for the benefits of the intervention as other aspects may be, such as the acceptability or cost-effectiveness of the treatment (Wykes and Spaulding, 2011).

One of the main differences among the different programs available refers to the explanatory focus of the mechanisms of neurocognitive recovery and the way to manage the deficits. These approaches are not specific to schizophrenia, but rather have already been applied in other neurological disorders such as acquired brain damage:

■ *"Restoration"* attempts to repair the neurocognitive deficits directly by the repeated use of exercises under the premise that cognitive deficits may be restored by stimulation. The remediation techniques developed within this focus are based on the repeated performance of exercises designed to regain the activation of the brain circuits and strengthen some basic processes.

■ The *"compensatory techniques"* do not attempt to restore the impaired cognitive skills but rather attempt to compensate or save the deficit by means of the use of alternative strategies, modifications in the environment, and the use of external aids such as environmental supports and prostheses, since this approach is based on the principle that cerebral mechanisms and cognitive processes may be recuperated.

■ The third approach, *"optimization,"* starts from the idea that not all the damaged cognitive processes are lost, but rather that their efficiency is diminished, and thus it aims at potentiating the performance of other cognitive processes which remain intact to guarantee function. Ideally, CR should combine these three approaches.

In relation to the above, Wykes and Reeder (2005) proposed the term *remediation*, since this does not necessarily imply a restoration to normality, which the term *rehabilitation* would imply.

Similar to the presence of different explanatory models of the mechanisms of recovery, different theoretical models of remediation have been developed, mainly from cognitive psychology, which we will briefly describe to provide better comprehension of the bases of CR. These models include, for instance, the model of limited capacity and the model of the activation threshold. More detailed information on each of the models may be found in some excellent CR manuals, such as those by Penadés and Gastó (2010) and Muñoz Céspedes and Tirapu Ustarroz (2001), both in Spanish, or that by Wykes and Reeder (2005).

Our program is based on applying the neurocognitive–behavioral model in an approach to the difficulties in functioning that bipolar patients present, as will be seen in the next chapter. The approach adopted is mainly compensatory; this has a sound basis in the "functional adaptation" approach supported by Luria (1963), but more importantly it reflects the current state of the evidence base relating to clinically significant functional improvements.

Neurocognitive–behavioral model

This model of cognitive–behavioral remediation involves both neurocognition and psychosocial aspects, combining neurological as well as neuropsychological aspects of behavioral therapy and those of cognitive psychology. With regard to the neurological aspects, this model considers the localization and the physiological sequelae of brain damage. From the neuropsychological perspective, this model is fostered by the definition of cognitive deficits and cognitive functioning from the different neuropsychological tests. At the same time, this model borrows behavioral-type interventions from behavioral therapy. Lastly, from cognitive psychology this model uses the idea of the possibility of neurocognitive change by means of control of the functioning itself. Therefore, CR should be understood as an intervention aimed at reducing functional problems and promoting integral remediation, considering the context of the individual and combining cognitive intervention strategies together with other pharmacological, behavioral, and psychosocial approaches. This focus requires an interdisciplinary approach and the joint work of several professionals.

Taking this perspective into account, the cognitive paradigm of *information processing* provides a theoretical framework that explains CR as a process of cognitive–behavioral intervention that has the objective of neurocognitive recovery and a reduction in the associated psychosocial disability, as mentioned above. Within this paradigm, knowledge is explained as the product of a successive series of cognitive operations that transform sensory information. The information undergoes a series of transformations until it reaches the final stage, the time at which the cognitive act is produced. These are *bottom-up* models. However, these models are also combined with *top-down* models in which the superior functions influence the processing of information at lower levels. There must be an attention filter to regulate the quantity of relevant and irrelevant information the subject receives from the environment (Broadbent, 1977). The relevant information is transformed into an icon (like an instant photo) which remains temporarily active in the iconic memory. This information is later encoded from the information available in the memory, thereby providing an additional significance beyond its simple physical and material properties. After this codification the information is ready for processing at another level. The quantity of information that can be kept in the short-term memory (or working memory, operative memory) is limited. Thereafter, the information may be stored in the long-term memory, depending on the subject's previous experience with this type of information, the motivation, and environmental conditions. If this information is stored in the long-term memory it can be recalled in the future by the processes of free recall or retrieval. At the same time, it can be recalled and used by the so-called frontal functions.

The neurocognitive deficits can therefore be explained when dysfunctions are produced in any phase of general processing – for example, an anomaly in the attention filter or an anomaly in the transfer of the encoded information to the long-term memory. The cognitive deficits which schizophrenic patients may present have been described using this model.

Another important characteristic of information processing is *serial functioning*, that is, the cognitive functions are related to each other. Thus, for example, an alteration at the attention level, which is a very early process, leads to alterations in subsequent processes such as information codification and consolidation. Nonetheless, other models were later proposed in which, despite the attention function being a system with limited capacity, different information can be processed simultaneously or "in parallel," provided that the limit of system capacity is not exceeded (Kanheman, 1973). This model led to the idea that cognitive demand increases with increasing complexity of the function, and if we add tasks until the limit of our capacity is exceeded, they are performed incorrectly.

However, within the paradigm of information processing we can also find the model of *parallel processing*, that is, different cognitive processes may occur simultaneously during the performance of simple tasks. Thus, the information acquired, encoded, stored, and recalled is not produced linearly but rather the different units of a network are simultaneously interconnected. These are the neuronal and computational models (automatic processing/controlled processing).

It should also be taken into account that the processing of information is carried out in a system of limited resources, resources which may focus on a single task or be divided into different cognitive processes. The characteristics of the task and the level of difficulty determine the distribution of the resources, going from automatization in simple tasks to a major controlled processing effort in which the use of a larger quantity of resources is necessary. However, at the same time the individual processing capacity may vary based on the physiological activation and other organic factors. Again, this model of limited capacity has been used to explain the cognitive deficits in schizophrenia (Penadés *et al.*, 1999; Vargas and Jimeno, 2002). The objective of interventions aimed at improving cognitive performance is, therefore, to diminish the demand of the task, facilitate the automatization of certain cognitive processes, or increase the processing capacity.

Apart from the paradigm of information processing, at a neuropsychological level another basic, key concept in CR is that of *brain plasticity* or *neuroplasticity*, which describes the capacity of the brain to modify its neuronal connections and networks; in other words, the possibility of transformation. This plasticity is considered the biological foundation on which the remediation of lost cognitive functions caused by a brain lesion is based. It allows functional restructuring of the damaged system, and of other areas not affected by an injury, so that these can partially assume the lost functions. It is known that traumatic and genetic factors, pharmacological treatment, environmental conditions, and other unidentified etiological processes can affect these connections, and it has also been suggested that therapeutic and pharmacological conditions can stimulate neuroplastic processes towards recovery. Nonetheless, it should be borne in mind that most of the results are derived from animal models (Wykes and Spaulding, 2011).

Training techniques

The different CR therapies are based mainly on the use of some training techniques. One of the techniques adopted in most of the programs is *"errorless learning,"* in which the therapist acts as a personal trainer who accompanies the subject in the learning of all the stages of performing the task, reducing the possibility of committing mistakes, with the aim of impeding error making during the learning process. As the subjects advance in their learning, they achieve greater skills and feel more confident, and the support is gradually withdrawn. Another technique used is *"self-monitoring."* This may be used in different ways; the basis of the technique is the use of internal language as a mediator of behavior: verbal instructions as reminders, self-instructions, or cues. It has been observed that this technique improves the performance of executive functions, although to the detriment of other tasks of lesser difficulty that depend more on speed than precision. Another prevalent technique is *"scaffolding,"* in which the therapist provides the guidelines until the subject is able to perform the task without difficulty. The therapist helps the patients in those skills which are beyond their possibilities, always requiring a minimum effort by the patients so that they feel neither bored nor overwhelmed.

Programs based on "practice and exercises" produce greater effects in improving cognition, while those using the learning of certain strategies produce greater effects on functioning. These latter programs work on memory and executive functions, teaching methods such as codification and grouping strategies (*chunking*) to facilitate recall or problem-solving techniques.

Intervention programs in psychosis

Before briefly describing some of the principal intervention programs mainly used within the setting of schizophrenia, it is worth remembering the 13 principles of remediation proposed by Prigatano (1999):

■ The clinician should begin the intervention focusing on the subjective and phenomenologic experience of the patients, to reduce their frustrations and confusion and to involve them in the remediation process.

■ The profile of deficit of the patient is a combination of cognitive traits and premorbid personality together with the neuropsychological changes produced by the brain damage.

■ Neuropsychological remediation is aimed at both the superior brain alterations and the management of interpersonal social situations.

■ Neuropsychological remediation helps the patients observe their own behavior and learn about the direct and indirect effects of the brain damage. This helps to better manage the catastrophic reactions and the choice of objectives and goals.

■ We do not completely know the relationships among cognition, personality, and emotion. This implies a partial understanding of certain questions of neuropsychological remediation.

■ We know little about the retraining of cognitive function, since the nature of these functions is not well known. However, we can establish some treatment guidelines for cognitive recovery.

■ Psychotherapeutic interventions are often an important part of neuropsychological remediation. They help the patient and relatives manage personal losses better. It is a highly individualized process.

■ Work with these patients produces emotional reactions in both relatives and therapists. Adequate management of these emotions is important, since it may influence the treatment of the patient.

■ Each remediation program should be dynamic, with constant change, permanent development, inexhaustible creative effort, and constant review of the scientific literature.

■ Failure to identify patients susceptible to successful treatment creates distrust and damages the credibility of the technique.

■ Alterations in awareness of the deficit are not sufficiently considered, and are often misunderstood and underestimated.

■ Competent, innovative planning is focused on adequate comprehension of the mechanisms of recovery and of the models of functioning and patterns of impairment.

■ Remediation of patients with impairment in high-level cognitive functions requires the use of scientific and phenomenologic evidence. Both are necessary to maximize patient recovery and adaptation.

The following **intervention programs** make up part of the wide range of possibilities in the field of schizophrenia, or in psychotic disorders more generally, and currently have empiric support.

Integrated psychological therapy (IPT) (Brenner *et al.*, 1994). This was the first program to include CR in a group format, and it was specifically designed for patients with schizophrenia. In addition to the cognitive elements being the main objective of the treatment, training in social skills is also included, with the aim of improving social behavior. Integral psychological therapy follows a hierarchic process which works with five subprograms from the most elemental to the most complex processes: cognitive differentiation, social perception, verbal communication, social skills, and interpersonal problem solving. Its efficacy in neurocognition and psychosocial functioning has been demonstrated, improving the codification skills and executive functions of the patients as well as their level of personal autonomy and social relations, in addition to observing permanence in this improvement.

Cognitive enhancement therapy (CET) (Hogarty and Flesher, 1999a, 1999b; Hogarty and Greenwald, 2006). This therapy combines a CR module with another on social cognition. The objective is to provide the subjects with experiences of cognitive enhancement through tasks performed with computer support, teaching cognitive strategies and experiences of socialization leading to advancement in social behavior. A part of the program is developed with tasks on the computer together with another patient and a therapist, and the tasks related to social cognition are carried out in a group. With regard to the content of the neurocognitive module, training is done in aspects of attention, memory, and problem solving. The tasks of social cognition include exercises of categorization, assessment of affect and of social contexts, resolution of social dilemmas in daily life, tasks of abstraction of ideas of news, and, lastly, starting and finishing conversations. The premise behind this program is that cognitive dysfunction represents a delay in social learning, a learning process developed from infancy to adulthood, and is thus a level of associated disability.

Attention process training (APT) (Sohlberg et al., 1994). This program is based on the premise that an improvement in attention is possible with the practice of exercises requiring the use of the different neurophysiological processes implicated in attention. The program is structured in a series of exercises that activate the neuronal circuits related to sustained, selective, alternative, and divided attention with four different packages of tasks: cancellation tasks, audio CDs, mental control tasks, and tasks of everyday life. It is applied individually, and not all patients should undertake all the modules, but rather it can be adapted to the individual characteristics of each patient.

Frontal executive program (F/E) (Delahunty and Morice, 1993). This program is carried out individually with pencil and paper. It has three modules which may be applied, depending on the deficits present in each patient: cognitive flexibility, working memory, and planning.

Cognitive remediation therapy (CRT) (Wykes and Reeder, 2005). The theoretical formulation of Wykes & Reeder's CRT represents a reformulation of the F/E with some overlap with CET. This program emphasizes metacognition and the use of techniques such as errorless learning and scaffolding. After developing cognitive strategies it aims at generalizing to daily life by problem solving, which involves the use of working memory, planning, and cognitive flexibility. The program is carried out in individual sessions.

Neuropsychological and educational approach to remediation (NEAR) (Medalia and Herlands, 2002). This program is found within evidence-based interventions, and thus its efficacy has been demonstrated in a number of well-controlled studies. It has one part with individual work (computer) and another part with group work. It uses cognitive–behavioral techniques to improve neurocognition and is based on a learning process. That is, the exercises are within a context that promotes interest in learning, facilitates the acquisition of the content, and promotes intrinsic motivation through the contextualization and personalization of learning, in addition to taking into account the process of generalization to real life. It is fundamentally fostered by learning methods based on the use of strategies.

Metacognitive skill training for patients with schizophrenia (MCT) (Moritz and Woodward, 2005). Metacognitive training (MCT) is a manualized cognitive intervention for patients with psychosis (it does not distinguish between affective and non-affective) with the objective of transferring knowledge of the cognitive biases/errors and providing corrector experiences. Among the problematic thinking styles recognized as potential contributors to the development of delusions are an increased self-serving bias (module 1), a jumping-to-conclusions bias (module 2 and 7), a bias against disconfirmatory evidence (module 3), deficits in theory of mind (module 4 and 6), overconfidence in memory errors (module 5), and depressive cognitive patterns (module 8). The main objective is to facilitate a reduction in symptoms and protect against relapses; however, basic cognitive dysfunctions, such as attentional problems, are not the subject of the program.

Neuroscience-informed cognitive training (Vinogradov et al., 2012). This is based on the notion that the brain can adapt throughout the lifespan to salient experiences by representing the relevant sensory and cognitive/affective inputs and action outputs with disproportionately larger and more coordinated populations of neurons that are distributed (and that are interacting) throughout multiple brain regions. It also implies that the impaired brain is capable of adaptive plastic change despite its underlying neuropathology, but that the magnitude of global improvement driven by any remediation method will be limited by the weakest link in the interacting neural systems. This neuroplasticity-based model addresses some of the limitations found in earlier remediation research, and proposes three important issues for consideration in the design of successful cognitive training for impaired neural systems.

One group of experts in neurocognitive remediation considers that several of these programs may be suitable as interventions for investigation by means of clinical trials (Keefe *et al.*, 2011). Nonetheless, some characteristics have been identified as being desirable for CR programs in schizophrenia, including the following:

■ Multiple sessions with learning, practice, and beginning to automate new cognitive skills.

■ Emphasis on increasing self-efficacy and intrinsic motivation.

■ Training manuals for clinicians who carry out the intervention, demonstration videos.

■ Demonstration of efficacy through measures of cognition and/or functioning.

Despite the different theoretical positions underlying the design of the various CR programs and the use of different techniques, at the base of all of these positions we can identify a common emphasis on the need for practice by the patients in order to achieve satisfactory performance, to prevent forgetfulness between consecutive sessions, and, from a neuroscientific perspective, to develop neural plasticity (Wykes and Spaulding, 2011). A common term in the literature on neuropsychological remediation – that of *generalization* – refers to the capacity to apply the principles and skills learned in the remediation sessions to daily life situations. Training based on strategies also uses practice, under the premise that generalization in the use of strategies through tasks will probably have a greater effect on future learning and the transference of this training. Thus, better generalization is required when the initial learning is carried out using different types of tasks in different situations similar to those used in real life (Rougier *et al.*, 2005). The concept of *contextualization* refers to the fact that if the material is presented within a practical utility and is related to real-world activities, it will be more useful for the subjects (Medalia and Choi, 2009).

Cognitive remediation should be developed in small steps (such as in the case of scaffolding and errorless learning) so that the participants can perceive a feeling of self-efficacy and can improve while also increasing the possibility of transferring this improvement into their daily lives. Likewise, if the patients perceive a task as being useful, their expectations are greater, and this fact will also be related to a greater perpetuation of the learning. This indicates that CR should be presented within a framework of personal goals, and that the tasks in the program should be clearly related to these objectives (Wykes and Spaulding, 2011). *Personalization* refers to this adaptation of the learning activity so that it converges with the subjects of interest to the subject in question; that is, the activities should be attractive, motivating, and interesting for the subjects so that they wish to continue participating in the intervention and can appreciate the relevance of each of the tasks performed. The establishment of a connection between the CR program and the objectives applied to the real life of the patient, such as in work, social life, or autonomy in daily tasks, is one possible way of establishing the relevance and utility of participation in these programs. Thus, a contextualization of cognitive tasks and the personalization of the learning process will probably lead to greater acquisition of cognitive skills, an increase in intrinsic motivation, and greater perception of self-efficacy (Medalia and Choi, 2009).

Cognitive remediation in bipolar disorder

The rapid development of investigations in affective disorders has demonstrated qualitatively similar cognitive deficits to those of schizophrenia, albeit of lesser magnitude, in other affective disorders such as bipolar disorder. It has therefore been suggested that cognitive remediation could also have a potential effect on individuals with some type of affective disorder.

Nonetheless, investigation in this field has been less developed, and there is still a long way to go. Most of the studies have been carried out in mixed samples including affective patients along with schizophrenia and schizoaffective disorders, making it difficult to draw conclusions. To date, only five studies have been undertaken in purely affective patients, and only one of these looked at bipolar patients (Deckersbach et al., 2010). The results of this study indicate that an improvement in psychosocial and occupational functioning may be achieved by an intervention focused on both cognitive and residual depressive symptoms (Fuentes-Dura et al., 2012). This focus also considers the subdepressive symptomatology, since it has been observed that this symptomatology has a close relationship with difficulties in global psychosocial functioning. Nonetheless, in this specific case, it should be taken into account that the beneficial effects of neurocognitive remediation may be confounded with mood improvement.

Despite the investigations coinciding in that more studies of CR in bipolar patients are needed, there is just one publication. Thus, at present we can only speculate as to the potential benefits of this intervention centered on unipolar and bipolar patients. The fact that the use of CR in affective disorders is still in its infancy provides the opportunity to learn from previously developed experience in the field of schizophrenia (Anaya et al., 2012). Nevertheless, it should be taken into account that, as mentioned previously, the cognitive deficits in schizophrenia patients are usually of greater severity than those presented by bipolar patients, and thus the programs aimed at schizophrenia patients may not be suitable for bipolar patients, because they are too simple and provide insufficient motivation for participation, leading to poor adherence (Fuentes-Dura et al., 2012).

More recently, a study protocol for a randomized controlled trial including 40 bipolar patients has been published by Demant et al. (2013) but results have not yet been published. In addition, a study of personalized cognitive training in unipolar and bipolar disorder was conducted in Prague, and findings have recently been published (Preiss et al., 2013). In this study, computer training was used and significant changes were found in the intervention group ($n = 15$) compared to the control group ($n = 16$) with regard to self-reported depressive symptoms and dysexecutive symptoms reported by a caregiver.

Chapter 3

Functional remediation in bipolar disorder

Introduction

According to data from the World Health Organization, bipolar disorder occupies the sixth place among the most disabling diseases (Murray and Lopez, 1997; Vieta and Gasto, 1997; Catalá-López *et al.*, 2013). Numerous investigations have demonstrated functional impairment in bipolar patients in comparison with both healthy individuals and unipolar patients (Kessler *et al.*, 2006; Parker *et al.*, 2007). Despite the great variability among patients, most (from 30% to 60% of bipolar patients) may present some type of functional impairment (Huxley and Baldessarini, 2007). This functional impairment may be prolonged, and may even be present during the periods of euthymia (Strakowski *et al.*, 1998; Fagiolini *et al.*, 2005; Tohen *et al.*, 2005; Goetz *et al.*, 2007; Rosa *et al.*, 2008). It is known that more than half of the patients do not recover previous functioning after an affective episode; in general only 40% of patients recover the grade of premorbid functioning during the periods of clinical remission (Tohen *et al.*, 2006; Delbello *et al.*, 2007). The difficulties in obtaining functional remission seem to be associated with disease progression; psychosocial adjustment is more preserved in patients with a first episode than in those with more chronic disease, with treatment being more effective in patients in the earlier stages of the disease (Tohen *et al.*, 2010).

A number of longitudinal studies have shown how functional recovery is much more complicated than clinical remission. One European follow-up study showed that 64% of patients achieved remission two years after an acute episode, but only 34% also achieved functional recovery; that is, they recovered the level of functioning prior to the onset of the disease (Haro *et al.*, 2011). In another follow-up study, it was found that 98% of the patients obtained symptomatic recovery at two years. However, only 38% achieved satisfactory functional recovery (Tohen *et al.*, 2000). In an eight-month follow-up study, Strakowski and colleagues (2000) observed that almost all of the patients presented persistent impairment in at least one of the areas of functioning studied and fewer than half achieved adequate functioning in three of the four areas assessed.

The factors involved in functioning remain unclear. According to several studies there is a direct correlation between the severity of the affective symptoms and the grade of functional impairment. Indeed, depressive symptomatology has the greatest impact on psychosocial functioning (Coryell *et al.*, 1998; Altshuler *et al.*, 2006; Kessler *et al.*, 2006; Delbello *et al.*, 2007; Judd *et al.*, 2008). These results are especially important, because many patients present depressive symptoms during most of their lives (Judd *et al.*, 2005). On the other hand, the rates of functional impairment are quite similar to the number of patients with neurocognitive dysfunction (Martino *et al.*, 2009). As noted in Chapter 1, neurocognitive impairment constitutes a central element of bipolar disorder, confirming the association between cognitive performance and psychosocial functioning. Several recent studies have found an interrelation between neurocognitive impairment and functioning in bipolar patients similar to that described in schizophrenia patients (Martínez-Arán *et al.*, 2007; Bonnín *et al.*, 2010).

One of the impaired areas of functioning found in these patients is the occupational area, in which a diminishment has been observed in productivity, with a greater number of days lost over one year and elevated unemployment rates (MacQueen *et al.*, 2001; Simon *et al.*, 2008). With respect to interpersonal relationships, one study carried out by our team reported serious difficulties in maintaining satisfactory sexual relationships, an increase in family and social conflicts, and reduced participation in social activities (Rosa *et al.*, 2009). With regard to family interaction, the quality of the relations among family members may affect the grade of psychosocial functioning and increase the number of relapses (Hammen *et al.*, 2000; Yan *et al.*, 2004).

How can we evaluate functioning?

The concept of functioning is complex and involves different aspects, including the capacity of work and study, the capacity to live independently, the capacity to enjoy leisure time, and the capacity to share life with a partner (Keck *et al.*, 1998; Strakowski *et al.*, 2000; Zarate *et al.*, 2000). Investigators traditionally measure one or two elements of functioning without taking all the others into account. The measurements of functioning used in this disorder vary greatly from one study to another; indeed, few measurements have been used by more than one investigator (MacQueen *et al.*, 2000; Altshuler *et al.*, 2002; Dean *et al.*, 2004).

Functioning may be measured by several scales, the most commonly used being the multi-dimensional scale for the evaluation of global activity (GAF). This is a hetero-administered tool that assesses the global functioning of a patient along a hypothetical continuum of health–disease. The higher the score, the better the level of activity. One of the frequent criticisms of this scale is that some of its operative criteria incorporate symptoms, mixing them with discapacity (First *et al.*, 1997; Altshuler *et al.*, 2002; Martínez-Arán *et al.*, 2007). Other scales used are the Social Adjustment Scale, the Life Functioning Questionnaire, the Short Form SF-36, and the WHO-DAS. Most of these scales require quite a long time for administration and were not designed specifically to evaluate functional alterations in bipolar disorder.

In response to the need for a simple, easy-to-use tool to evaluate functioning in bipolar disorder we developed the FAST scale (Rosa *et al.*, 2007) (see Appendix 1). This is a highly reliable tool to evaluate the objective difficulties presented by patients in psychosocial functioning, an area which has also demonstrated sensitivity to changes in both the short and the long term (Rosa *et al.*, 2011). The scale was designed taking into account the most frequent difficulties found in bipolar patients. It only has 24 items, allowing its integration into daily clinical practice as well as its use in investigation. It provides a total global score of discapacity (from 0 to 72) and another six subscores for the six domains of the scale: autonomy, occupational functioning, cognitive functioning, financial issues, interpersonal relationships, and leisure time. The efficacy of the intervention may therefore be measured in terms of global improvement in general, but also in terms of improvement in each specific domain.

Functional recovery is one of the questions which remains to be solved in the treatment of bipolar disorder. In clinical practice there is a need to reduce the impact of the disability of bipolar patients in order to diminish the suffering and the cost of this disease. Cognitive remediation (CR) is widely used in patients with schizophrenia and psychosis. However, as described in Chapter 2, only five studies have to date been performed on CR in affective bipolar and unipolar patients, and of these, only one was focused on bipolar patients (Deckersbach *et al.*, 2010). The number of bipolar patients included was not specified in the other studies. The sample sizes in these studies were small, ranging from 2 to 18 patients, and the duration of the interventions was from 8 to 48 weeks. In general, the CR programs used cognitive measures pre- and post-intervention to evaluate the efficacy of the program.

3

Chapter

How was the functional remediation program developed?

We developed the program in the Hospital Clínic de Barcelona, with the main objective of treating not only neurocognition but also functional impairment in bipolar disorder. We have coined the term *functional remediation* to refer to an innovative intervention focused especially on the recovery of the psychosocial functioning of the patients through training in the use of neurocognitive skills applied to daily routines. The functional remediation program is the first approach carried out in the field of bipolar disorder with the aim of improving the psychosocial functioning of these patients. The program is based on a neurocognitive psychosocial focus including modeling techniques, role playing, self-instructions, verbal instructions, and positive reinforcement, together with metacognition. It includes education on cognitive deficits and their impact on daily life, and provides strategies to manage the cognitive deficiencies in the different cognitive domains, mainly attention, memory, and executive functions (Martínez-Arán et al., 2011). The family is also involved in the process to facilitate the practice of these strategies and for reinforcement. It is important to combine different theories, methodologies, and approaches in order to improve not only the knowledge but also the functioning of these patients, given the complexity and the severity of bipolar disorder.

Inclusion and exclusion criteria

- The target group for this intervention involves patients with bipolar disorder, although patients with bipolar-type schizoaffective disorder may also benefit from the program.

- The patients included in the program must have been euthymic for at least the last three months.

- If a patient does not attend a session he/she is given the material corresponding to that session. If he/she does not attend five or more sessions of the program, and if the absenteeism is not justified, the patient is excluded from the group. If the reason for the absence is a small relapse not requiring hospitalization and the patient has missed fewer than five sessions, he/she may rejoin the group.

- The functional remediation program is aimed at people from 18 to 60 years of age; it is not directed at first episodes of the disease, but in case of cognitive and functioning difficulties these patients may be included in the program.

- The patients must be receiving psychiatric follow-up, and must be taking the appropriate pharmacological treatment.

- Patients receiving electroconvulsive therapy (ECT) should be excluded until the treatment has been completed in order to be able to benefit from the intervention.

Efficacy of the functional remediation program

The efficacy of this program has been demonstrated in a recent controlled clinical trial comparing three treatments: psychoeducation, functional remediation, and pharmacological treatment only (standard treatment) (Torrent et al., 2013). Ten Spanish centers participated in this multicenter study, recruiting a total of 268 patients. These centers are members of CIBERSAM (Centro de Investigación Biomédica en Red de Salud Mental: the Spanish psychiatric research network) and have extensive experience in the investigation and clinical management of bipolar disorder. With the aim of guaranteeing the reliability of the interventions, the coordinating center, the Hospital Clínic de Barcelona, organized three meetings for training in the assessment and performance of the two active interventions (functional remediation and psychoeducation).

An outline of the sudy design is shown in Figure 3.1. The patients were randomized into the three study arms, stratified by sex, age, and educational level. Pharmacological treatment was

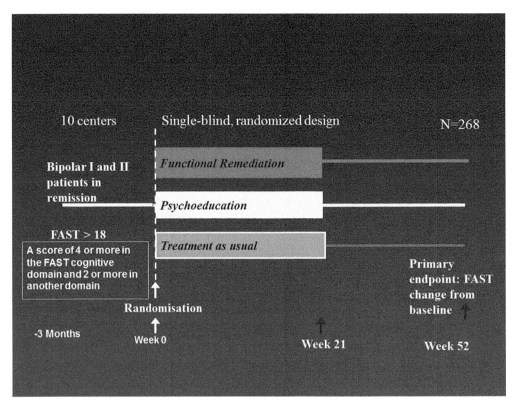

Figure 3.1 Study design.

prescribed to the three groups according to local clinical guidelines. The psychoeducation program applied was created in our Bipolar Disorders Unit in the Hospital Clínic de Barcelona, has proven efficacy, is internationally recognized, is endorsed in the clinical guidelines for the treatment of bipolar disorder (Colom *et al.*, 2003, 2006), and has been translated into several languages.

Relevant sociodemographic and clinical data were collected, and the functional assessment was carried out using the Functioning Assessment Short Test (FAST) (Rosa *et al.*, 2007; see Appendix 1). To study the neuropsychological variables, the tools listed in Appendix 2 were used, based on a review of the literature and the selection of the most documented (Spreen and Strauss, 1998; Lezak *et al.*, 2004) and most frequently used tests in bipolar disorder (Martínez-Arán *et al.*, 2000; Goodwin and Jamison, 2007). The clinical, neurocognitive, and functional assessments were repeated at the end of the interventions. The criteria for discontinuation in the study were as follows: failure to attend five or more sessions of the intervention groups, hospitalization or severe relapse, or withdrawal of consent.

The main measure of efficacy consisted of changes observed in psychosocial functioning post-intervention and at one year, as assessed with the FAST, with respect to the baseline evaluation. Thus, once the intervention was completed, the patients were again assessed at a clinical, functional, and neuropsychological level.

The results showed an improvement in the functioning of patients participating in the functional remediation group compared with those who did not receive any intervention other than pharmacological treatment, based on the mixed model of repeated measures ($p < 0.001$), as shown in Figure 3.2. In addition, patients undergoing the functional remediation program achieved significant improvement in occupational and interpersonal or social functioning compared to those with only the usual pharmacological treatment (Figure 3.3). The efficacy of the functional remediation intervention program was maintained at one year of follow-up. Six-month follow-up results have been published (Torrent *et al.*, 2013), and the one-year results have recently been submitted for publication. At the one-year follow-up, autonomy

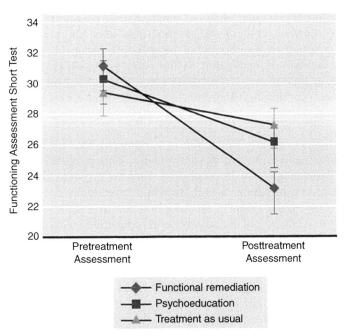

Figure 3.2 Changes in functional impairment scores before and after intervention in patients with bipolar disorder.

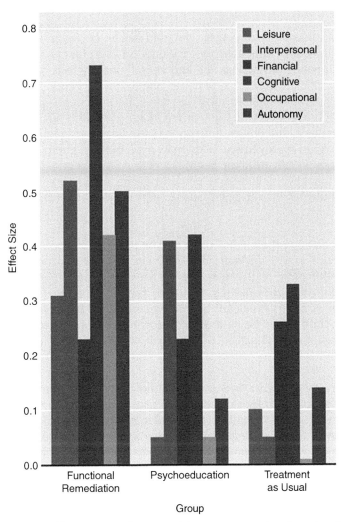

Figure 3.3 Within-group effect sizes in functional improvement, by domain of the Functioning Assessment Short Test.

was improved in those patients who received functional remediation. Although no significant improvements were seen on neurocognitive measures after six months, improvements in verbal memory were found in the functional remediation group at one year, so the use of cognitive strategies is likely consolidated in the long term, which may result in a better functional prognosis. Verbal memory has been recognized to be a mediator between subsyndromal symptoms and functioning (Bonnín et al., 2014), so improving memory may lead to improving functioning.

The functional remediation program therefore is a promising tool for achieving improvement in functional performance in euthymic bipolar patients. This program is not a simple training course to improve neurocognition, but rather it aims to provide tools for the patients to manage the difficulties and problems of real life which affect daily functioning. It is important to reduce the impact of bipolar disorder on daily functioning within an ecological framework to thereby increase the wellbeing of the patients and reduce the costs and social burden of this disease.

The functional remediation program may improve aspects related to work functioning, increasing economic autonomy and reducing financial dependence. Indeed, approximately 5% of the patients obtained work or improved their occupational performance after the intervention. The interpersonal relationships improve partly by means of the group effect, which facilitates relating to other people, but it should be taken into account that aspects related to memory, strategies for codifying information, and social skills (recognition of emotions, assertiveness) are emphasized. The patients often have to interact to carry out the exercises or tasks, potentiating the feeling of self-confidence.

With respect to neurocognitive changes, the differences between the three groups were not statistically significant, although the patients in the functional remediation group showed better performance on the learning and verbal memory tests, gaining advantage from the strategies of semantic encoding. Nonetheless, the following cannot be ruled out: the effect of practice as well as other factors must be taken into account, such as that this trial's inclusion criteria required a certain level of functional disability but not necessarily neuropsychological impairment. The object of functional remediation is general functional improvement, not just cognitive improvement. This may explain why improvements in functioning were larger and more significant than neuropsychological changes. The results suggest that even though some cognitive deficits may persist, patients exhibit greater ability and are able to employ more strategies to cope with these deficits in daily life after having received specific training.

The functional remediation program has proven to be effective in improving the functioning of patients with bipolar I and II disorder, especially in the areas of occupational and social functioning. A combination of pharmacological treatment and functional remediation in patients with relevant difficulties in their daily life could improve the functional prognosis of persons with bipolar disorder. Although the intervention could be implemented at an individual level, the group format may be more effective, not only from an economic point of view, representing an important saving of time, but also because it facilitates interpersonal interaction.

We know that patients with bipolar disorder present deficits in some domains of social cognition (theory of mind and emotional processing) even in phases of euthymia (Colom, 2012; Samamé et al., 2012). The deficits in social cognition may lead to poor social functioning, and it is therefore imperative that mental health professionals reach a greater consensus and improvement of methods used in the assessment of the domains of social cognition in bipolar disorder. It is also important that functional/neurocognitive remediation programs should include interventions directed to improve social cognition.

Patients obtain benefits that improve their functioning from the functional remediation program, but these effects would most probably be more prolonged and could be generalized to different settings of daily life and to other areas of functioning if the training could be continued, supervised, and monitored by a therapist on completion of the intervention. In this regard, booster sessions every three months or at least twice a year would be very helpful in order to maintain practice and positive results, to review the content, to determine whether the learning has been consolidated, and to establish whether the patients have integrated the new guidelines into their everyday routines.

Chapter 4

Functional remediation program: sessions and content

Structure of the program

The 21 sessions that constitute the intervention are divided into five blocks or modules (Table 4.1).

Module 1 contains the first three sessions, devoted to training on neurocognitive processes. In one of these sessions the relatives of the patients are included in order to explain the objectives of the intervention and clarify any questions related to neurocognitive deficits and their implications in daily life. In addition, the relatives are recommended to encourage the patient to attend the sessions and to do the homework, potentiating their autonomy whenever possible. Session 2 deals with educating or training the patient in neurocognitive deficits. There may be some dysfunctional beliefs and prejudices related to patients' neurocognitive deficits which make them feel anxious or embarrassed. The main objective of this session is to explain the nature of the disability and the relationship between disease progression and neurocognitive dysfunction. Session 3 is related to the preceding session, explaining that positive and negative factors that may interfere with neurocognitive impairment and functioning are elements over which they can exert a certain control. A further aim of session 3 is to contradict some of the myths which they may believe, and thereby to help the process of de-stigmatization.

Module 2 consists of sessions 4 and 5, and this is the point at which the real training in neurocognitive functions begins. These sessions are devoted to the different types of attention: selective attention, sustained attention, and divided attention. The theoretical basis is explained and training is done with different exercises.

Module 3 includes sessions 6 to 11 and contains the block devoted to memory. Not only are internal strategies practiced (association, organization, categorization, etc.) in these sessions, but the option of using external aids (diary, clock alarms, information and communication technologies [ICTs], for instance) is also explained. One of the sessions of this block is dedicated to reacquiring the reading habit. The main objective of this session is for the patients to acquire or reacquire this routine in their lives. To do this the patients are asked to read a book, starting in session 10. The reading is organized as a number of chapters each week, and the patients must respond to a series of questions proposed by the therapists to evaluate their level of comprehension. The book becomes one of the homework tasks. The questions and their difficulty are adapted to the educational level of the group.

Module 4 contains the block on executive functions and includes five sessions (12 to 16). During these sessions, the nature of these functions is studied in depth and activities are carried out within an ecological setting to learn how to plan, program, manage time, adapt to unforeseen events, and establish priorities, alongside training in effective problem solving.

Module 5 is the last block and includes sessions 17 to 21. These sessions are related to improving communication, interpersonal relationships, autonomy, and the control of stress. Finally, in the last session, a recap of what has been done is made, and the patients evaluate the intervention.

Table 4.1 The structure of the functional remediation program: 21 sessions, in five modules

MODULE 1: TRAINING ON NEUROCOGNITIVE PROCESSES
1. Introduction to functional remediation. The role of the family. Enhancing practice and reinforcement.
2. What are the most common cognitive dysfunctions in bipolar disorder?
3. Factors influencing cognitive impairment: myths and realities.

MODULE 2: ATTENTION
4. What is attention? Strategies for improving it.
5. Strategies to improve attention and their application in daily life.

MODULE 3: MEMORY
6. What is memory? Strategies for improving it.
7. Memory: the use of a diary and other external aids.
8. Internal strategies to improve memory.
9. Other mnemonic strategies and their application in daily life.
10. Reading and remembering.
11. Puzzles: retrieving information from the past.

MODULE 4: EXECUTIVE FUNCTIONS
12. Executive functions: self-instructions and self-monitoring.
13. Executive functions: programming and organizing activities.
14. Executive functions: programming activities, establishing priorities, and time management.
15. Executive functions: problem-solving techniques.
16. Executive functions: solving problems.

MODULE 5: IMPROVING COMMUNICATION, AUTONOMY, AND STRESS MANAGEMENT
17. Managing stressful situations.
18. Training in communication skills.
19. Improving communication.
20. Improving autonomy and functioning.
21. Final session: review of useful strategies.

Organization of the sessions

The intervention consists of 21 weekly sessions of 90 minutes in length, each of which is divided into four parts:

(1) The first 15–20 minutes are devoted to discussing the tasks of the previous session and any difficulties encountered in performing the task or any doubts regarding the previous session.

(2) After discussing the homework, the theory part of the session is initiated, in which the central theme of the session is explained (20–25 minutes).

(3) The next part is devoted to practical tasks, doing the exercises proposed and providing tasks for the following session. The practical part consists of pencil-and-paper exercises, some of which are individual, others in pairs or small groups, lasting 40–45 minutes. This is the most important part of the session. The format of the exercises facilitates cooperation and cohesion among the members of the group while indirectly working on interpersonal relationships and improving communication. The objective of these exercises is to adapt them to the difficulties of the real world so that each patient can find the best strategy to use to improve his or her functioning in daily life.

(4) The final part of the session involves an explanation of the homework and an examination of the key points of the session. At the beginning of each session and after discussing the tasks we collect the patients' individual homework, and this is returned, corrected and with comments (if necessary), in the next session. It is recommended that the patients should not do all the homework on the same day but rather divide it up through the week. It is very

important that we keep up to date with this work, because receiving the corrected home-work with comments each week acts as positive reinforcement to maintain the patient's motivation to continue working at home.

Material and therapy room

The basic material for implementing the program requires a computer and a projector to show the slides and a whiteboard for taking notes. There are two different sources of material available online, material for the therapists and material for the patients. Both include a PowerPoint slide set. The therapists' slides should be shown during each session, and the slides for the patients should be printed (three per sheet, allowing space for notes) and handed out to the patients at the beginning of each session. As an example, we have inserted some of these slides within this chapter to illustrate and clarify the content of the sessions.

In the therapist material there is also a document containing questions and possible answers on the book *The Little Prince*, which the patients are encouraged to read as homework from session 10 onward. In the patient material, in addition to the slides, you will also find the homework dossier for each session, to be handed out as well, and a collection of handouts summarizing each session, to be delivered during the session. This handout is also available within every session in this chapter in the section *Material for the patient*, but the online version is intended to be easily printed out, in order to facilitate the development of the session.

Depending on the session, complementary material is needed as specified. A chronometer will be necessary in almost all sessions.

The exercises proposed in each session must present graduating difficulty, in order to easily maintain the motivation of the patients.

The therapy room must have sufficient space for 10–12 people, and insofar as possible it should have little outside noise. The chairs should be placed in a circle to promote group interaction.

Therapist training

The therapists should be psychologists with a background in neuropsychology, and they should have experience both with patients with bipolar disorder and in carrying out group sessions. These are some general guidelines to be taken into account by the therapist:

■ Before each exercise, explain the objectives to be achieved, to increase patient motivation.

■ Emphasize that what is important is the learning, and the exchange of useful strategies for everyday life, rather than the final result of the tasks.

■ Provide clear instructions, and ensure comprehension by all members of the group.

■ Encourage active participation, to increase motivation, interpersonal communication, and group cohesion.

■ The therapist should adopt a directive role, and should encourage participation, as this has a positive reinforcing effect. Encourage the group to analyze contributions.

■ Politely but firmly reject comments not related to the exercises or tasks, as these may interfere with the group dynamic.

■ Apply cognitive–behavioral techniques: role play, positive reinforcement, verbal instructions, self-instructions, metacognition guidelines, modeling, etc.

■ Propose work to be done at home, to reinforce and generalize what has been done in the session.

■ Address the patient by name before asking a question.

■ Repeat information, aiming to minimize any silences.

■ Attempt to create a friendly, open environment. Introduce the exercises and homework as a game, ensuring that they are interactive.

■ Listen to others without judging or criticizing, showing respect toward their opinions and their different responses.

■ All the members of the group should have the opportunity to participate, so that no one person dominates the debate. To achieve this, establish turns.

■ Do not rush. Some sessions may have more tasks or exercises, or may result in greater participation by the members of the group. In this case some of the tasks may be carried out in another session in which more time is available, or can even be proposed as homework.

Module 1. Training on neurocognitive processes

This module is essential, because its objective is to provide basic information to the patient and his or her relative(s) concerning the cognitive deficits that may be present in persons with bipolar disorder, and to promote awareness of the difficulties that these deficits may cause in day-to-day activities.

Although this part of the intervention program is called the training or education module, we refer to some aspects of metacognition, since, in this module, we intend to help patients (and their relatives) become aware of issues related to their own cognition (thinking about thinking – metacognition) and understand the factors that may explain or influence their performance. Metacognition refers to any knowledge or cognitive process which supervises or controls cognition itself; in other words, it includes the knowledge patients have of their own cognitive capacities and the regulation of their cognitive activity. The metacognitive processes allow people to identify mental states, to reason about them, and to attribute cognitive processes to themselves or other persons.

Therapists cannot take it for granted that all patients presenting these types of cognitive difficulties are aware of them, or of the repercussions they may have on their daily functioning, whether at a social, occupational, or academic level. Most patients presenting cognitive difficulties are quite aware of their difficulties, but a group of patients, perhaps a relatively small minority, may not be conscious of their own deficits and their impact at a functional level. At the same time, we also find patients who are aware of their cognitive limitations but do not realize that those limitations may be secondary to bipolar disorder and the group of factors involved that can help us to explain some of the cognitive deficits.

On the other hand, in clinical practice we sometimes find patients who are not sufficiently aware of these difficulties, and some of their relatives or persons close to them may be even less aware. Nonetheless, in general, the relatives and persons close to the patient are usually reliable informers who provide clinically relevant information to healthcare personnel. The bipolar disorder may, on occasions, lead to some concerns among those close to the patient, who may think that the person uses the fact of having the disease as an excuse for stopping doing certain tasks about the house, forgetting appointments, etc. Relatives or close friends probably better understand or accept the difficulties patients experience when they have an episode (manic or depressive), but they may not understand why they continue acting the same way when asymptomatic or in remission, and may, for example, report that their relative shows a certain indifference or laziness in doing some everyday tasks. On the other hand, it should also be taken into account that some relatives may adopt an attitude of overprotection, interpreting all the reactions of the patient as if they were a product of the disorder and not allowing them to develop their own autonomy. Therefore, knowing the points of view of relatives and patients separately may be important, since thereby we may sometimes detect significant differences between the information provided by the relatives and that provided by the patients themselves. An assessment of the extent of the disagreement between the two sources, if any, may constitute an essential element in establishing the level of self-awareness of the limitations that is experienced by the person with bipolar disorder.

This module is placed first to allow both patients and relatives to become aware of the cognitive difficulties that may be presented, but also because this module introduces some key concepts that will be more extensively developed in later sessions. For the patients, this psychoeducational work is important as a means of promoting knowledge related to the cognitive limitations they may present, paving the way for de-stigmatization and allowing the limitations to be acted upon. In addition, it provides a useful way of helping them to understand their problems, while also giving them greater autonomy and preparing the ground for providing a set of cognitive techniques and strategies in later sessions. For the relatives, it is important to understand that many of the difficulties presented by the patient originate from the cognitive problems rather than from an attitude, and that participation in an intervention of this type may allow modification of some of these aspects and directly influence the overall functioning of the person with bipolar disorder.

It is therefore important to achieve an intermediate point at which acceptance of the disorder is incorporated, restructuring the expectations of the psychosocial functioning of the individual and, in turn, encouraging the performance of tasks to potentiate that person's autonomy without, of course, overburdening the patient.

Session 1. Introduction to functional remediation; the role of the family; enhancing practice and reinforcement

Objective

The main objective of this session is to make contact with a relative or someone close to the patient, to provide information regarding the cognitive deficits that people with bipolar disorder may present, the impact these may have on daily life, and the role which they, as relatives, may play in helping them in an attempt to potentiate their autonomy.

It is often difficult for relatives to understand that the patient presents difficulties in carrying out some everyday tasks, such as not remembering that they should do something they were asked to do, forgetting to take their medication, etc., when the patient is not in an affective episode (mania or depression). Therefore, it is of great importance to make the relatives aware of the cognitive difficulties the patient may experience even when in remission. In this session the main objective of the functional remediation groups is explained, along with the role that relatives can play, and, lastly, relatives are given a series of guidelines to follow when interacting with the patient, designed to minimize the cognitive problems while at the same time potentiating greater autonomy of the patient.

Likewise, the involvement of the family in the process of functional remediation may be essential to motivate the patient to continue with the intervention, in addition to reinforcing the knowledge acquired and the progress made by the subject, and stimulating the practice of the new strategies that the patient acquires through the course of the intervention.

Session procedure/guidelines for the therapist

Prior to setting up the groups the patient is informed that this session is exclusively for the relatives, and authorization is requested for a maximum of two relatives per patient to attend. Although this is the first session, each center may schedule this session later on, for example when we are already somewhat familiar with the patients after the second or third session. Normally a different day of the week is chosen, being flexible so that the relatives can attend and the patients do not miss the day scheduled for their session.

During this session, the relatives are introduced to the possible cognitive deficits that their relative with bipolar disorder may present. They are given a detailed explanation of each of the principal cognitive domains, with some examples of each so that they may be more easily identified, and they receive an explanation of why these deficits exist. It is emphasized that not all patients present the same pattern of cognitive difficulties, nor do they have the same level of severity of difficulties or impact on daily life.

COGNITION and bipolar disorder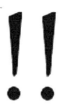

- Not all patients have all these difficulties.

- Some have deficits in some areas (e.g., problems with attention and memory) but not in others.

- Other patients have a combination of the different types of cognitive dysfunction.

- A cognitive study is necessary for each patient.

Session 1 slide 15

Thereafter a brief explanation is given concerning the factors that may negatively influence cognition, and that may potentially be controllable, as well as the factors that have a positive influence.

Cognitive deficits in bipolar disorder

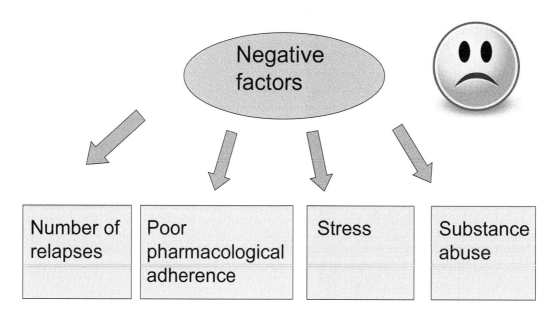

Session 1 slide 16

Cognitive deficits in bipolar disorder

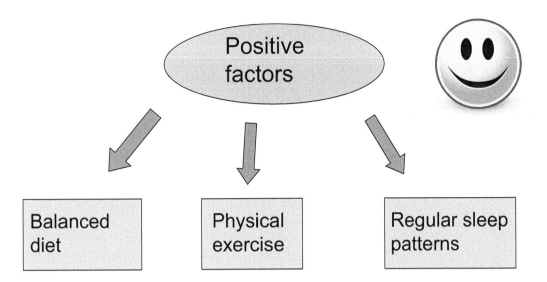

Session 1 slide 17

One part of this session that is likely to be of great interest to relatives is the guidelines concerning how they can act to help the patient with these cognitive difficulties.

Role of the family, and guidelines

- Motivate the patient to carry out the tasks set in the group sessions, and reinforce him/her.
- Give clear messages and instructions, to reduce the amount of information to remember.
- Reduce distractors.
- Give the patient the necessary time to complete the activity.
- Encourage patients to do things for themselves. Provide incentives to use external aids: anything that facilitates memory and organization (diaries, calendars, etc.).
- Realistic expectations.

Session 1 slide 18

As an in-situ task, towards the end of this session, time is given for the relatives to have the opportunity to voluntarily comment upon the most common cognitive problems observed in their relatives, the factors that they consider may influence these deficits, and the repercussions on daily life.

At the end of the session a summary of the key points is made. Ask one of the participants to read them aloud. This procedure is repeated at the end of each session.

Material for the relatives

People with a bipolar disorder may present difficulties, for example in maintaining attention, in learning and remembering information, and in organizing or planning everyday activities, among others. These problems are frequent and affect approximately 30–60% of the patients to a greater or lesser extent. These difficulties are commonly known as cognitive deficits; they may be increased during episodes of mania and depression, although some deficits may persist when the patient is without or practically without symptoms.

One of the essential factors negatively influencing cognition in these patients is the **number of relapses**. The greater the number of episodes of the disease the patient experiences, the more evident the cognitive difficulties will probably be. Thus, it is fundamental to prevent relapses to avoid the damage that these may cause in cognitive functions. For example, if you notice changes in mood state, a reduction in the number of hours of sleep or the need to sleep, or hyperactivity, it is important to contact the psychiatrist to avoid a new relapse.

Poor treatment adherence, that is, incorrect medication or not taking medication, increases the risk of relapse, and this is associated with further cognitive problems. Nonetheless, a patient with cognitive deficits may also often have difficulties in correctly following the medication schedule, generally because the patient forgets to take the medication.

Stress factors produce important hormonal changes leading, on one hand, to a greater risk of relapse and, on the other, to cognitive deficits. In addition, use of **toxic substances** has a negative impact on cognitive function in bipolar patients, making it important to avoid their consumption.

Some positive factors related to cognitive function include **adequate and balanced nutrition,** avoiding restrictive diets or the missing of meals. **Physical exercise** is useful, avoiding an excessively sedentary life. Walking and programmed activities may help those not interested in sports. Finally, **regular sleeping habits** are very necessary, not only to prevent relapses but also to improve cognitive functioning; eight hours of sleep are recommended daily.

Through the rehabilitation groups we hope the patients will manage their cognitive problems better, will be aware of the difficulties, and will have a series of strategies to manage these difficulties. The objectives are essentially for the patient to make greater and better use of external aids (diary, notebook, mobile phone organizer, etc.) and other strategies to promote greater autonomy in a range of everyday tasks or activities.

The role of the family is basically:

- To promote the practice of the strategies that the patient acquires in the rehabilitation groups, and to reinforce them positively for their use.

- To allow the patients to do everything they are able to independently by themselves (bathing and personal care, shopping, collaboration in household tasks, being responsible for some administrative tasks, etc.) while, on the other hand, taking into account the patient's present mood state. If the patient is depressed this should not be confused with apathy, and difficulty in carrying out and performing activities should not be confused with indifference and laziness.

Expectations regarding the changes must be realistic. We must reinforce behaviors that improve or are more adaptive but ensure not to generate conflicts or arguments with respect to aspects that could be improved. Frustration may sometimes appear when time passes and the patient is unable to reestablish previous functioning.

Bipolar disorder may sometimes lead to uncertainty and, in the long term, overload among the relatives, who, on occasions, may not know how to act. In these cases it is important to seek out help in support groups and to receive more information from associations or from the psychiatrist and/or psychologist (family groups, psychoeducation).

In the rehabilitation sessions the patient will learn new strategies which should be applied to situations in daily life, and it is therefore important to motivate the patient. It must be remembered that the strategies will not make the memory problems disappear, but they will help with better management of the difficulties. In the last sessions of the program the patient will acquire more skills to confront stressful situations and solve problems.

The limitation of the number of activities the patient performs reduces the possibility of learning from experience. The therapists will ask the patient to perform tasks that can successfully be done, with a progressive rise in the level of difficulty of the tasks. The increase in the level of difficulty is approached as a challenge, and success in performing the task will encourage the patient to continue making an effort and to resume activities that were previously enjoyed.

Some points to follow:

- Reduce the quantity of information to remember, giving messages and clear instructions.

- Provide simple instructions (checklists, including the steps to follow, e.g., for the use of a new apparatus, an electrical device, or a computer program).

- Give them the necessary time to complete the activity (e.g., ten minutes instead of five for taking a shower, to plan the clothing to wear the next day, or to make breakfast).

- Encourage the use of external aids (diary, alarm, mobile phone organizer, etc.).

- Encourage patients to autonomously do the tasks they are able to do by themselves (e.g., do not call them to remind them to take the medication when an acquired strategy such as an alarm or post-it may be used; do not have the patient wait for a member of the family to get home from work before going shopping when it can be done alone, using a list).

- Encourage the use of self-instructions and self-monitoring (what must be done, choose the strategy, carry out the chosen behavior, and assess the final result).

Key points

- Cognitive problems are very common in bipolar patients. In these group sessions the patient will learn new strategies that may be applied in everyday situations.

- Promote patient autonomy, encouraging the patient to do all that he or she is able to do independently, without forgetting the mood state at that time.

- Encourage the practice of the strategies that the patient acquires in the rehabilitation groups, motivating the patient to continue performing homework tasks and reinforcing the advances made.

Session 2. What are the most common cognitive dysfunctions in bipolar disorder?

Objective

It can be said that this session is based on three objectives. Firstly, contact is made with the group and the rules for the group sessions are explained to all the members. This first session is crucial to establish good contact between the patients and the therapists and to explain some rules for good group functioning, which will serve as an aid to establish a good working environment and facilitate the participation of the members of the group. Secondly, the main objectives of the intervention are explained to the participants. Lastly, education related to the main cognitive deficits that persons with bipolar disorder may have is started. In this section, the biological bases of the cognitive deficits present in bipolar disorder are explained, and some key concepts, which will be more extensively developed in subsequent sessions, are introduced.

Session procedure/guidelines for the therapist

Before beginning the session, the room should be prepared, placing several chairs in a circle facing the screen where the slides will be shown.

After the introduction of the therapists present during the session, the next step is to present the program, the objectives of the program, the duration of the session (21 weekly sessions of 90 minutes each), and the methodology of the intervention.

Afterwards, the norms of good group functioning are explained in detail. It is pointed out that if the rules are not followed, a member of the group may be expelled:

- *Confidentiality*. Neither the identity of the other members of the group nor what they discuss during the sessions is to be commented upon outside the group. However, the content of the session and the explanations given by the therapists or the tasks performed may be commented on, and there is no prohibition regarding patients meeting outside the sessions.

- *Attendance*. To obtain the most benefit from the group and facilitate group feeling, it is obligatory to attend all the sessions. Any patient who does not attend five sessions without good reason will be expelled from the group.

- *Punctuality*. This is a basic principle for correct development of the session. A systematic lack of respect for this norm will also mean expulsion from the group.

- *Respect*. The opinions of the members of the group must be respected. No mocking, laughing, or negative criticisms regarding the comments of a member of the group will be accepted. Repeated lack of respect will also result in expulsion from the group.

- *Participation and practice*. It is highly recommended to actively participate in the sessions, making and responding to questions and carrying out the tasks given during the sessions and at home. A participative attitude will help everyone to gain the greatest advantage from the group.

Following the explanation of the rules, we present the objectives of functional remediation. It is useful to ask each participant about their expectations at the time of accepting to participate in this type of intervention. If any member of the group seems to have an expectation that does not match what a functional remediation program is, this is the appropriate time to establish the real objectives of the program. It is important to clearly explain what the intervention consists of, and to emphasize that it is not a psychoeducational program on bipolar disorder. Most of the patients know the objective of the intervention since it will usually have been explained previously. It will most likely be relatives who are not familiar with it, or for whom it is not clear what this type of intervention is based upon.

Goals of functional remediation

- Learn to **better manage** cognitive problems.

- Training in the use of different **techniques and strategies** to minimize the impact of cognitive difficulties, such as the use of external aids (diary, mobile phone, etc.).

- Increase patient **autonomy** in some tasks or activities in daily life.

Session 2 slide 3

The final major section of this session consists of an introduction to the main cognitive deficits that people with bipolar disorder may experience. We clearly and concisely explain some basic related concepts, such as what the limbic system is, neurons and the way they communicate, and the hippocampus, among others, to facilitate greater comprehension of the biological basis of the cognitive deficits present in bipolar disorder. In this section we can introduce and explain new concepts such as executive functions, which is a concept not usually known by most patients. Then we can explain the relationship between cognitive deficits and daily functioning, that is, the repercussions that these types of difficulties have on tasks carried out in daily life.

Limbic system

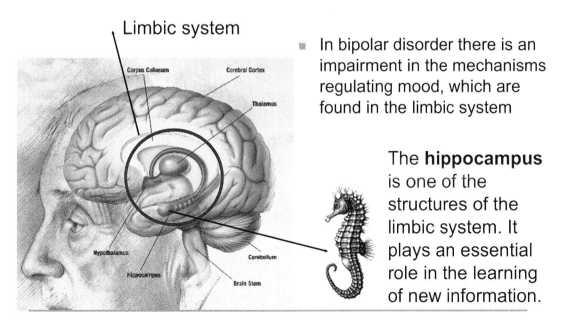

Limbic system

Corpus Callosum
Cerebral Cortex
Thalamus
Hypothalamus
Hippocampus
Cerebellum
Brain Stem

- In bipolar disorder there is an impairment in the mechanisms regulating mood, which are found in the limbic system

The **hippocampus** is one of the structures of the limbic system. It plays an essential role in the learning of new information.

Session 2 slide 6

Neurocognitive disturbances and functional outcome

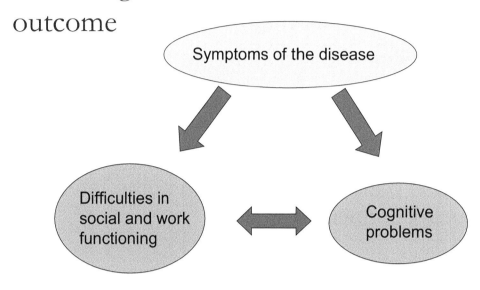

Session 2 slide 9

We then introduce the members of the group, asking each one of them to introduce themselves by name. In the first round both the patients and the therapists should introduce themselves. After the individual introductions, a reminder round is made in which each of the patients says his or her own name and those of the other members of the group. If a patient does not remember the name of a specific member, that person should help by giving a clue. The therapists also participate in this naming round.

Lastly, we explain the homework to be done and ask a volunteer to read the key points aloud.

Homework

■ The homework for this session is for the patients to list the cognitive difficulties that they most frequently experience (frequent forgetting, distractions, etc.) and what they think are the causes.

Material for the patient

Norms for good group functioning
■ **Confidentiality**. The group activity should not be discussed outside the group, nor should the identity of the members or what is discussed during the sessions be made known. However, the content of the session may be discussed with regard to the explanations given by the therapists or the tasks performed, and there is no prohibition regarding patients meeting outside the sessions.

■ **Attendance**. To obtain the greatest benefit from the group and facilitate group feeling, all the sessions must be attended. Any patient who does not attend five sessions will be expelled from the group.

- **Punctuality**. This is a basic principle for correct development of the session. A systematic lack of respect for this norm will also mean expulsion from the group.

- **Respect**. The opinions of the members of the group must be respected. Mocking, laughing, or negative criticism of the comments of a member of the group will not be tolerated. Repeated lack of respect will mean expulsion from the group.

- **Participation and practice**. Active participation in the sessions is highly recommended, including asking and responding to questions and carrying out the tasks set out during the sessions and at home. A participative attitude will help everyone to gain maximum advantage from the group.

Cognitive difficulties

In psychiatric consultations patients with bipolar disorder often complain about problems of concentration and memory. Until recently it was believed that these difficulties were present during the episodes of mania and, particularly, in those of depression. However, we have progressively become aware that cognitive problems or deficits go beyond the boundaries of the episodes and sometimes persist even when the patient is asymptomatic or practically euthymic (stable). Since these complaints are very common, investigations are increasingly being performed in relation to these problems in bipolar patients and how they affect everyday functioning.

We will begin by clarifying what cognitive or neurocognitive functions are. This concept refers to functions related to attention, memory, speed of information processing, and the executive functions which, basically, imply the organization and planning of our responses and behavior, the control or inhibition of behaviors (which may be inadequate), and decision making, as well as the capacity for abstraction and reasoning. This seems complex because we are talking about many new terms which we will be working with little by little over the coming weeks. We will have enough time to become familiar with the most important of these terms. Therefore, cognitive deficits refer to difficulties in one or more areas of the functions mentioned above. In the following sessions we will explain in greater detail the functions in which the most common alterations are found and how to improve the difficulties by following some schedules and strategies.

In general, in the case of bipolar disorder, difficulties are found in three of the areas mentioned above: attention, memory, and executive functions. Each of us may experience greater difficulty in one area or another, and thus there are individual differences.

The difficulties are due to the production of a series of changes in our brain which are translated into cognitive problems. It must be taken into account that our brain has limited space and weighs approximately one kilogram and a half. Neurons are basic elements of the nervous system. Biologists have calculated that our brain contains around one hundred million of these nerve cells, which communicate through chemical and electrical signals. There are also different molecules called neurotransmitters which act as mediators to transmit the information from one neuron to another (acetylcholine, GABA, dopamine, adrenaline, glutamate, etc.).

In bipolar disorder there is an alteration in the mechanisms which regulate the mood state, which, simplifying a little, are basically found in the limbic system. In addition to being responsible for regulating the emotions, the limbic system, also called the emotional system, is a part of the nervous system that has a fundamental role in learning and memory.

The hippocampus is one of the structures of the limbic system which plays an essential role in the learning of new information. The information is systematically passed through the hippocampus to be analyzed and coded and is thereafter distributed to different zones of the brain. Therefore, the memory does not reside in any specific place, but rather is widely distributed throughout the brain and is supported by associative cerebral structures responsible for establishing links between the different elements making up a memory.

General functioning

In addition to the symptoms of bipolar disorder, the cognitive deficits influence how a person relates to their immediate environment. For example, difficulties in remembering things or following a conversation, or in adequately organizing oneself, may make it difficult to follow a "normal" rhythm of functioning and may, on occasions, reduce social relationships and diminish work performance. In other cases, the disease itself and often the cognitive deficits may lead to a prolonged situation of work leave, or even make the patient unable to work or have to carry out another simpler type of work with less stress or requiring less concentration or memory. However, the reduction in the level of activity and social interaction may, in the long term, have negative consequences on our cognitive functions, since with inactivity we do not use neural connections and this hinders the functional recovery.

In later sessions we will provide strategies to compensate for some of these difficulties and, more generally, to improve everyday functioning.

Key points

- In bipolar disorder we often find difficulties, particularly related to attention, memory, and executive functions.

- These difficulties may affect everyday functioning, for example in learning and remembering information, maintaining attention, and organizing ourselves to carry out various tasks.

Session 3. Factors influencing cognitive impairment: myths and realities

Objective

The main objective of this session is to present a series of factors that may potentially both negatively and positively influence cognition. It is emphasized that the patients have some control or are able to manage some of these factors. In general terms, we can say that this session covers the key aspect of psychoeducation in bipolar disorder related to cognitive deficits, since the key is to be aware of the factors involved in the course, evolution, and prognosis of the disease. However, attention must be focused on the factors that especially affect the cognitive function, with the final objective of understanding that a reduction in relapses as far as possible and an improvement in the course of the disease will indirectly help to prevent the cognitive and functioning problems in the medium to long term. The factors to be worked on are those which may be controlled by the patients, and for which they may therefore assume some responsibility.

In relation to the factors that may influence cognition, we work on some "myths and realities" that may lead to erroneous beliefs and cognitive distortions. The purpose of this section is to discover the beliefs and attitudes of our patients, to understand what prejudices they have, to know what point we are at, and, if necessary, to explore some aspects in depth to avoid the continued holding of certain misconceptions by some of the patients which, at certain times, could lead to them making poor decisions (for example, abandoning pharmacological treatment in the belief that the treatment is the cause of the cognitive difficulties).

4

Chapter

Session procedure/guidelines for the therapist

This session starts by collecting the homework and discussing it briefly.

Next the factors that may negatively influence cognition in persons with bipolar disorder are presented, along with what aspects can be controlled or improved.

Negative factors

- ▩ Number of relapses
- ▩ Substance use
- ▩ Sleep disorders
- ▩ Poor treatment adherence
- ▩ Stress

Session 3 slide 2

These key issues will make the patients aware of the factors that affect the course of the disease as well as cognitive functioning, with the aim of avoiding, insofar as possible, a greater number of relapses and emphasizing the importance of adherence to pharmacological treatment – avoiding substance abuse, which could worsen the course of the disorder as well as the cognitive functions per se. In addition, the importance of regular sleep habits and avoiding or learning to better manage situations of stress is underlined. When discussing toxic substance consumption we can also explain some relevant aspects related to the intake of substance usually not considered harmful in bipolar disorder, such as coffee and alcohol.

A clear, concise, brief explanation is given of the vicious circle presented by greater vulnerability to stress, greater risk of relapse, the changes these represent at a cerebral level, the cognitive difficulties, and their impact at a functional level.

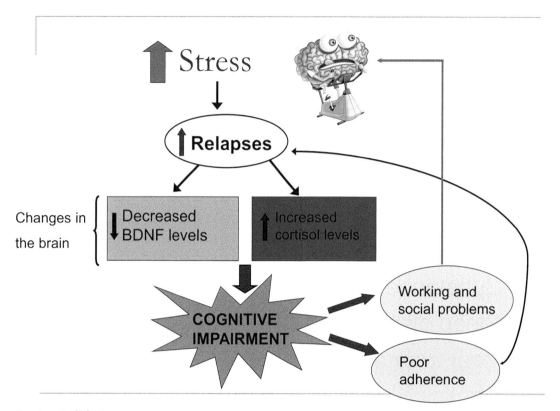

Session 3 slide 3

Thirdly, the positive factors which may influence and which we may potentiate to improve cognition are explained, as is the importance of maintaining an adequate and balanced diet, an adequate level of physical exercise/activity, and regularity in sleep (sleep hygiene). Overall, we discuss the importance of regularity in our habits and of attempting to maintain a healthy lifestyle, since this has a positive effect not only on the bipolar disorder itself but also on cognitive deficits.

Thereafter we show a series of slides of "myths and realities," first asking the patients what they believe or what their opinion on this is. Then we show them the other part of the slide explaining why this is a myth. As noted previously, some patients may have some erroneous ideas about the disease, which may make it difficult for them to recognize their problems, and may lead them to make inadequate decisions at certain times, so work on these aspects is beneficial.

As an in-situ task, time should be made to discuss the possible causes of cognitive difficulties with the group.

To finish, we should explain the homework to be done and ask for a volunteer to read the key points out loud.

Myths and realities

"The medication causes the cognitive deficits"

> Cognitive problems are generally a consequence of the disease itself. In fact, there is increasing evidence that medication such as lithium or valproate exerts a protective effect on neurons (neuroprotection). The same has been found for some antipsychotics and antidepressants.

Session 3 slide 8

Homework

■ Each patient is asked to list the tricks or strategies he or she uses for problems of concentration, memory, etc.

Material for the patient

Different factors may influence our cognitive functions (attention, memory, executive functions). Below we will see that some of these may be especially important because of their negative effect, and others may be positive. We will focus on those over which we have some control or management.

Negative factors
■ One of the essential factors with a negative influence on cognitive problems is the **number of relapses**: the more episodes of disease we have, the more cognitive difficulties we will probably have. In addition, it seems that manic episodes in particular have the greatest effect on the capacity for concentration and memory. Therefore, it is fundamental to prevent relapses to avoid the damage that these may cause to the cognitive functions. For example, if we notice changes in mood, a reduction in the sleep hours or the need to sleep, hyperactivity or racing thoughts, it is important to contact the psychiatrist to avoid a new relapse.

■ **Substance abuse,** including alcohol, may also have harmful effects not only on the mood state but also on aspects such as the memory, generating an inability to retain new information. Substance abuse or dependence may have adverse effects on attention and superior functions such as decision making or cognitive flexibility, in addition to seriously worsening the course of the disease. On the other hand, even caffeine may constitute a stimulant. It is not harmful in small doses but is dangerous if consumed in excess, causing insomnia and an increase in anxiety.

■ **Sleep disorders,** such as insomnia or interrupted sleep, may affect the mood state. In addition to producing irritability or excitation, on occasions, the patient may perceive greater memory failure. The psychiatrist will search for the best solution to this problem, and the therapy offered by the psychologist (sleep hygiene, relaxation techniques, etc.) will be very useful.

■ **Poor treatment adherence,** that is, incorrect medication or not taking medication, carries a greater risk of relapse, and this is associated with more cognitive problems. Nonetheless, it is also common for patients with cognitive deficits to have difficulties in correctly following medication schedules, generally because they forget to take it.

■ **Stress factors** produce important hormonal changes, carrying, on one hand, a greater risk of relapse and, on the other hand, cognitive deficits. During prolonged situations of stress the levels of cortisol are increased, while the levels of neurotrophic factors such as brain-derived neurotrophic factor (BDNF), which have a neuroprotective effect, are reduced – and this leads to changes in the functioning of our brain, affecting some cerebral structures such as the hippocampus, the amygdala, and the prefrontal cortex. These changes are translated into more or less persistent cognitive deficits.

Positive factors
■ **Adequate** and balanced **diet,** avoiding restrictive diets or missing meals (to be covered in later sessions).

■ **Physical exercise,** avoiding an excessively sedentary life. Walking and doing a programmed activity may be useful for those not interested in sports.

■ Sleeping nearly eight hours daily; this **sleeping regularity** is necessary not only to prevent relapses but also to improve cognitive difficulties.

Myths and realities
■ "The **medication** is the cause of the cognitive deficits." This is false. Most patients believe that lithium or other drugs produce the difficulties encountered. Although in some individual cases the drug or drug combinations required to improve or at least not worsen these deficits must be evaluated, in general the cognitive problems are the consequence of the disease itself. Research studies are increasingly providing data on the protective effect medications such as lithium or valproate, and even some antipsychotics and antidepressives, have on the neurons (a neuroprotective effect). The greatest risk is when the patient decides to stop taking the medication without consulting the physician because of the fear of developing cognitive side effects. It is preferable to consult with the specialist regarding this fear and allow the psychiatrist to adequately inform the patient as to possible options.

■ "The presence of attention or memory problems means that one is increasingly less intelligent." False. The **general intellectual level** does not vary, it is stable; one continues to be equally intelligent, despite experiencing more difficulties in concentrating or remembering things. In bipolar disorder the intelligence quotient (IQ) does not diminish with time.

■ "There is greater intellectual capacity during the **episodes of mania and hypomania.**" False. One may have the impression of having a greater facility to associate ideas, but the mechanisms of association are inefficient. Although patients may think they have a supermind, the truth is that symptoms such as distraction diminish the capacity to differentiate what is relevant from what is not. Thoughts may be so disorganized (e.g., a sensation of seeing several TV channels at the same time) that one cannot achieve adequate storage of information.

■ **"Cognitive impairment is progressive** and leads to dementia." False. There are deficits, but there is no evidence that these worsen over time. The risk of developing dementia in bipolar disorder is similar to that in the rest of the population.

Key points

■ Relapse prevention is important to avoid cognitive problems.

■ Aspects such as sleep hours, balanced diet, and the level of daily activity should be controlled to reduce cognitive problems.

■ The consumption of alcohol and other substances should be avoided, and taking the correct medication will help to improve the illness course and avoid cognitive difficulties insofar as possible.

Module 2. Attention

With this module the proper training in cognitive functions starts. Sessions 4 and 5 focus on attention as the basis for other cognitive functions. We explain roughly what attention is, the types of attention, and which aspects of daily life are interfered with by deficits in this area. Strategies are provided, to be worked through during the sessions and as part of the homework between the sessions. The main point is to place the emphasis on the importance of attention as a foundation for other areas of cognitive function, and the strategies acquired will be used in subsequent sessions. One such strategy consists of concentrating on one activity, such as a word search, or looking for differences between two images, or a mental calculation task, while having other elements of distraction in parallel, such as noise or background music. Part of the strategy involves taking breaks during attention-straining tasks, and limiting oneself to carrying out one task at a time rather than attempting to multitask a number of activities or initiate new activities before other activities are completed.

Session 4. What is attention? Strategies for improving it

Objective

This is the session in which the training and practice of strategies actually begins. We start with the cognitive domain of attention, since it is the basis of all the cognitive processes, intervening as a filter of environmental stimuli, deciding what stimuli are most relevant, and giving them priority through concentration. At the same time, attention is understood as the mechanism that controls and regulates the cognitive processes.

The different types of attention are explained: the most basic level corresponds to sustained attention; the next level is selective attention; and lastly the type of attention that implies the greatest difficulty is divided attention, which involves maintaining attention in two or more tasks at the same time.

Using examples, we explain everyday life situations in which attention problems play a role, such as losing the thread of a conversation, not remembering the name of an interlocutor, or difficulties in following the argument of a film or in reading a newspaper or novel. In this session the patients begin to put into practice some strategies to improve these aspects. In both this session and the next it is important to introduce an element to regulate the attention process, such as the verbal instructions necessary for correct execution of the tasks. At first the verbalization is external and explicit, but later it becomes internal and implicit, with self-instruction.

Session procedure/guidelines for the therapist

This session requires a small radio and chronometer.

Collect the homework from the previous session and briefly discuss it with the group (approximately 10 minutes). In this case the subject to be discussed is the tricks or strategies that the members of the group use to avoid memory and concentration problems. Encourage them to actively participate in explaining their experience. The tricks or strategies contributed by the patients themselves are often very welcome and useful for the rest of the group.

Supervision of the tasks by the therapists is very important to maintain patient motivation and to ensure that the homework is done, which, in turn, allows active participation in the group sessions.

Afterwards we initiate the theoretical part of the session, explaining the concept of attention by means of the metaphor of theater lighting. Another metaphor used to explain this concept is that of two torches, to learn to adequately control our attention.

What is attention?

- Attention is a brain function. Its purpose is to select between multiple stimuli reaching the brain simultaneously.
- A useful metaphor is the lighting system of a theater:

  - The lighting is selective and has a certain intensity, and the objects outside the illuminated field are ignored.

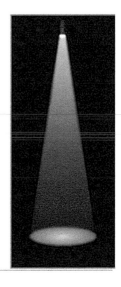

Session 4 slide 2

After explaining the three types of attention we start with the practical work.

Firstly, we do two rounds to consolidate the learning and remembering of the names of the group members: each participant gives his or her name and those of the rest of the group.

Then we begin working on sustained attention, testing how much information we can retain at once. The group is shown the winning numbers in a lottery for a short time (20 seconds) and is then asked to write down all the numbers they remember on a sheet of paper. It is important to ask them if they used any strategy to perform this task. If so, they are asked to share the strategy with the group. If no, they are offered some strategies to facilitate remembering (for example, ordering the numbers in increasing size, grouping the information, or associating the numbers with significant dates or ages of persons close to them). This same exercise is done with telephone numbers.

We then begin to work on selective attention, based on the same principle of remembering winning lottery combinations, but in this case with the radio on as a distractor. We should point out to the patients the difference in doing the tasks in silence and with the radio on, which requires selective attention.

To finish the session we propose some exercises such as word searches, looking for differences between two images, and mental calculation tasks ordered by degree of difficulty. Provide strategies for word searching. In this regard, we emphasize the relevance of cognitive stimulation, so that patients can use different options in everyday practice, such as Scrabble, playing cards, sudokus, etc., depending on their preferences.

We end the session by reading the key points aloud and explaining the homework.

Homework

To continue practicing at home we propose more word searches, looking for differences between two pictures, and more mental calculations. The group members are encouraged to continue doing such tasks on their own. For patients with computers, we can suggest some websites where these tasks can be found in order of difficulty. We stimulate the patients to incorporate exercises of this kind into their daily routines at home in the coming weeks. Based on the examples and tasks provided during the session, the patients will most likely feel more comfortable doing one type of exercise/task or another. They should be encouraged to continue practicing between sessions, and to maintain the habit even after the group sessions are over. Patients who read a newspaper can take advantage of the various puzzles and mental exercises that appear there. Praise should be given to participants who bring in material additional to the homework that they have worked on during the week.

Material for the patient

Attention is a cerebral function that allows us to persistently focus on a stimulus or carry out a specific activity. Attention is the basis of all the cognitive processes and is, therefore, not an isolated activity but rather intervenes in the processing of information, facilitating the working of all the cognitive processes, regulating and exercising control over these processes.

The right cerebral hemisphere is the hemisphere directly involved in attention. Many bipolar patients show attention difficulties, which are associated with problems in both work and social settings. Attention is produced in response to both auditory and visual stimuli.

Attention is a very broad concept, and for better understanding we have divided it into three levels or parts:

- ■ The most basic level of attention is that of **sustained attention**. This is defined as the ability to maintain attention on a specific activity – for example, listening to a conference, watching a television program or film and following the argument, reading the newspaper, concentrating on a conversation, etc.

- ■ The next level of attention, presenting greater difficulty, is so-called **selective attention**, which consists in concentrating on one activity while having other elements of distraction in parallel, such as noise or background music. In this case the information that is important must be filtered, as we attempt to focus our attention on what we really want. For example, being able to hold a conversation in a bar with loud music, crossing the street safely with the many visual and auditory distractions, attempting to listen to the television while hearing a heated argument between the neighbors or the siren of ambulances passing by.

- ■ The situation that presents the greatest difficulty is **divided attention**, which involves paying attention to two or more tasks at the same time – for example, watching our favorite television program while ironing clothes. Cooking also often involves several activities at once – while watching the eggs fry, we are cutting the bread . . .

One of the manifestations of attention problems is usually distractibility. When concentration problems are present, it is difficult to enjoy everyday activities such as going to the cinema, reading the newspaper or a novel for half an hour, etc. Or we may ignore some data that may be important in the context of a conversation, such as missing a sentence that is important to follow an argument or not remembering the name of the speaker. Sometimes the person begins to avoid situations for fear of not doing them well or because they are too complicated, leading to progressive social isolation and an increase in symptoms of depression. It may also be frustrating for the person to see how other people do not understand these difficulties well, interpreting the patient as absent-minded or having bad manners.

In the next two sessions we will undertake some group exercises to attempt to reduce the impact that these difficulties have on our daily lives. It is important to keep in mind that there are no magic solutions, but we will provide some tasks to do at home to consolidate the training.

Key points

- Attention is the basis of all the cognitive processes and allows us to persistently focus on a stimulus or on a chosen activity, such as reading or watching a film.

- Attention problems are associated with problems in both work and social situations.

Session 5. Strategies to improve attention and their application in daily life

Objective

This session is essentially practical. The objective is to consolidate the use of strategies for the management of the main deficits of attention. After reminding them of the main guidelines to take into account for working on attention, we start by practicing different exercises, individually and in pairs. Each patient should adopt the strategies and exercises which personally work best for them. Our objective is to propose a wide range of strategies, so that each patient can personalize them, adopting those that provide them with the best results.

Session procedure/guidelines for the therapist

After asking if there are any questions about the previous week, we collect the previous exercises and, depending on the time available, correct most of the tasks together. The tasks that cannot be corrected during the session are collected, to be returned, corrected, the following week.

Before starting the session we do a warm-up task working on mental calculation. In the first round we start with the number 32, and each participant in turn adds 5. In the second round we start at 80 and subtract 6 each time. The therapists generally also participate in the rounds.

We make a general summary of the guidelines to work on attention, such as modifying expectations, establishing rest periods during the activity, changing tasks at a pre-established time, using chronometers or alarms, rewarding ourselves (self-reinforcement) on finishing the task, taking notes, reducing distracting stimuli, using self-instructions, and focusing on "active listening."

The first task to carry out in the session is one called the *whole sentence*. Active, careful listening to each of the words read by the members of the group is very important in this exercise. Give out a card to each patient with a word belonging to a sentence by a famous writer or one we have made up ourselves. Each patient must recite the words the previous members of the group have read out, and then add the word on their own card, until the sentence is complete.

The second task for this session is the *sudoku*. This is a pastime that has become internationally popular in the past decade. The object is to fill in a 9×9 grid (81 cells), divided into 3×3 grids called "blocks," with the numbers from 1 to 9, starting with some cells already filled with numbers. Explain the rules of the puzzle and fill in the sudoku with the guidance of the therapist and the participation of the members of the group. Ask the group about the level of experience they have with this type of task, which involves visual attention as well as working memory. If possible, we can pair up the patients according to their experience with sudokus (suggestion: pair up one with experience with one without). Provide some online links at which sudokus of different degrees of difficulty can be found to practice at home.

We then work on visual attention through illustrations, providing guidelines to help focus attention, first globally (large torch), and then more focused on the most relevant details (small torch), screening or scanning the image with the instruction of formulating mental questions about the content of the illustration.

Homework

At the end of the session we explain the tasks to be done at home – for example, word games such as anagrams and incomplete words, as well as more "ecological" tasks, such as exercises calculating the change for purchases made, observing a room and the elements or details within it, noticing establishments while walking in the street or the position of products on the shelves of a supermarket.

Material for the patient

In this session we will work at a practical level with a series of exercises. Below we provide some guidelines and strategies that may help to improve attention and manage the deficits:

- Modify expectations, and give yourself a longer period of time for each activity, if necessary.

- Plan for breaks: the rest periods of an activity are important. If you see that your attention is diminished after 10–15 minutes, plan for a rest of a couple of minutes during which you may drink some water or do some relaxation exercises. A rest period of a few minutes every hour is recommended.

- Changing tasks at certain pre-established times may help to maintain your attention.

- Use an alarm or a clock.

- Use self-instructions to redirect your attention towards what you want to achieve.

- Give yourself a "reward" every time you finish a task (self-reinforcement).

- In general, information that is clearly of interest to us is remembered more easily, and therefore it is important to choose books or newspaper articles which a priori motivate us more.

- Nevertheless, even if what you see or hear is not of interest to you, attempt to identify and pay attention to the most relevant data.

- Practice active listening. Try to participate in the conversation of your interlocutor, for example, by asking questions to clarify doubts. This will help you to retain the information better and maintain your attention.

- Get used to not only talking but also listening, paying attention to "key" aspects of the person you are talking with, related both to tone of voice and to posture. This will help clarify the message.

- When reading an article, ask yourself what the main idea is, what this news means, what the opinion is, etc. In the beginning, it may be useful to underline the principal ideas in the text.

- Take notes, because writing helps us to visualize what we need to remember and to develop memory by means of the motor activity. Later revision of the information will also facilitate memory.

- Reduce external distractions as far as possible. Turn off the television if you want to read, and work in a quiet room. Make an effort, trying to ignore distractions. Change your surroundings if necessary.

- Establish routines to avoid situations that imply more than one task simultaneously. For example, avoid talking on the telephone while reviewing emails.

Key points

- The use of guidelines and strategies may be helpful in improving attention and managing cognitive deficits.

Module 3. Memory

Sessions 6–11 address memory. The steps in the process of acquiring and retrieving memory are impacted by the illness, and this module includes various exercises focusing on remembering visual and auditory verbal input, with several strategies to enhance encoding, storage, and retrieval of the information. The group of techniques promotes a more profound processing, elaborating the information so that it acquires a structure with more significance. The main techniques to be specifically explained are *association*, *categorization*, and *narration* or story. Other strategies provided are: restitution technique, rhythm and rhyme, repetition technique, method of loci. We will also work on some strategies that allow the reconstruction of information from the past, such as better organizing the memories with well-classified, ordered, and labeled photos, recordings, or videos of important events. The exercises in this module also include a reading task, where patients have to start reading a book and choosing a piece of news in the newspaper to track for several weeks. Before starting the tasks, we refresh memory techniques, such as reading aloud, taking brief notes, and using visual imagery in order to remember instructions and key points.

Session 6. What is memory? Strategies for improving it

Objective

The objective of the sixth session is to provide information to the patients regarding the concept of memory and its functioning, and to initiate the practice of strategies to improve it and reduce the impact of memory difficulties on their everyday routine. To illustrate the concept we will use the metaphor of memory functioning like a library in which the patient is the librarian in charge of classifying, labeling, and filing the books (adapted from the book *No Me Acuerdo* ["I don't remember"], Rafael Penadés and Teresa Boget, 1999).

Session procedure/guidelines for the therapist

We start the session by collecting the tasks from the previous session. We briefly discuss them out loud, asking if any difficulty was encountered (maximum of 10 minutes) or if there is any question or general comment about the previous session.

Before beginning the session we do two warm-up rounds (one in each direction) to work on mental calculation. For example, in the first round we start at the number 38 and each participant adds 7, and in the second round we start at 75 and each person subtracts 4.

We begin by explaining the three processes of memory – encoding, storage, and retrieval – and then the types of memory – sensory, short-term, and long-term.

The session contains visual imagery exercises, including one done in pairs in which the patients sit back to back to work on aspects of visual attention with respect to each other. They each have to make a brief description of the physical appearance of their partner and how he/she is dressed that day. This is done with no prior warning.

Another variant of the exercise may be for each participant to cover his or her watch and attempt to describe it.

4

Chapter

Visual imagery exercises

- Observe situations or people. Then, with your eyes closed, try to remember the details. For example, we can do an exercise: paying attention to the clothing of the person next to us and then trying to remember the details.

Session 6 slide 17

In another visual imagery exercise to be done in pairs, one of the two partners should explain what his or her bedroom is like, and then the other should make a drawing of it. Questions, displayed on a slide, can be used as a guide to help to visualize and remember the room. Having done this, the two partners should check the results together. If time permits, one of the two can voluntarily demonstrate the exercise to the remainder of the group. There is no exchange of roles in this exercise.

To continue working on visual attention and how this facilitates subsequent remembering, patients are shown an illustration of, for example, a well-equipped kitchen. The picture should be shown for one minute. The patients have to remember the techniques explained for focusing attention, making a global view of the most specific and relevant details, and formulating mental questions about the content of the picture (e.g., using the two torches).

As an option, a slide with questions referring to the picture may be shown. This picture should be projected for three minutes so that the patients have time to answer.

To end the session we hand out the homework dossier corresponding to this session.

Positive reinforcement of the tasks performed during the session is very important.

Homework

- The first task encourages the patients to continue practicing the visual imagery tasks explained during the previous session: notice the objects around them in the street; focus attention on the products on the shelves in a shop or supermarket; pay attention to the metro stops that remain before their destination, etc.

■ Ask how many patients use a diary-type resource to note the things they have to do, and if this resource is adequate. Also ask if they have access to technology such as a computer or mobile phone, as a potential resource.

■ It is useful to determine whether some patients use applications on their mobile phones such as Instagram, which allows original and different photographs of the environment to be used. Using such an application involves having to focus attention and notice details of the surroundings. In general, patients who use new technologies are more likely to share these strategies, and even devote time to teaching other interested members of the group how to use them. This reinforces the search and exchange of strategies that facilitate everyday functioning.

Material for the patient

Memory is a brain function that allows us to remember past experiences. There are various aspects to the concept of memory. On the one hand it refers to the image that comes to mind when we evoke a memory from childhood, while on the other hand it refers to abilities we have learned such as riding a bicycle or playing the piano, guessing a commercial from hearing only the jingle, remembering a friend, etc. Memory also includes knowledge that one has acquired – for example, the year in which World War II began, or the name of the artist who painted the *Mona Lisa*.

According to this pattern, there are different types of memory:

(a)   **Sensory memory** – by which we register information through the senses. The information registered by different auditory, olfactory, visual, tactile, and other stimuli accedes to the brain. Sensory memory has great capacity and brief duration.

(b)   **Short-term memory** – this type of memory produces temporary, fragile storage of information in the memory for 20–45 seconds, with a volume of 2–7 elements. After this, if the information is not reinforced and passed on to the long-term memory, it is lost.

(c)   **Long-term memory**: this is a memory store where the information we receive remains for a long time:
  (i)   **Episodic memory** – this is the fact of remembering things that have happened to us. It refers to particular events in our life such as past vacations, birthday celebrations, etc.
  (ii)   **Semantic memory** – this refers to our archive of general knowledge, whether it is cultural, such as the history of the country or lists of capital cities, or relates to other concepts such as multiplication tables.
  (iii)   **Procedural memory** – this is related to the ability to learn activities expressed behaviorally such as riding a bicycle, driving a car, or playing an instrument.

In general terms, verbal memory is localized in the left hemisphere of the brain, while non-verbal memory is situated in the right hemisphere. The objective is to discover which type of memory is more developed and attempt to use it to compensate for other less-developed types.

There are different stages in the process of memory:

1st   The information is registered, that is, it is perceived: we receive and process the information we wish to keep, through our senses (**encoding**).

2nd   The following stage is that of retaining the information: we store the information we have processed (**storage**).

3rd   In the last stage, we retrieve the information we have registered and stored beforehand (**retrieval**).

In other words, remembering something means first searching for and localizing it in our memory and then extracting it. In a figurative sense we could say that memory works like a library.

More than half of people with bipolar disorder show memory problems; they have difficulties remembering things that they have to do, lose objects, forget things, and have problems remembering the names of people, words, etc.

Recent research has studied the possible causes of this phenomenon, and it is recognized that memory problems are associated with factors such as the number of episodes (especially manic phases) and hospitalizations, not taking the medication correctly, etc.

In this session and the next one we will work together to provide strategies to reduce the impact of memory difficulties in our everyday lives. The strategies used will be both external and internal.

Key points

- Memory is a brain function that allows us to remember past experiences.

- Memory includes different aspects: evoking childhood memories, abilities learned, remembering an appointment, etc.

- The three stages in the memory process are: information encoding, storage, and retrieval.

Session 7. Memory: the use of a diary and other external aids
Objective

The objective of this session is to learn to manage external aids and optimize their use. By *external strategies* we mean instruments or tools with which we attempt to reduce the impact of cognitive deficits on daily life and compensate for some altered functions. It is important to "de-stigmatize" the use of these aids, normalizing their use and transmitting the concept of creating a personalized "tool box" that each patient will fill with the techniques and strategies that best help him or her achieve compensation for the impaired functions and improve daily functioning.

Session procedure/guidelines for the therapist

We start by getting the group to discuss the external strategies used. It should be taken into account that some patients will already have their own organization system. The objective is not to change this system but rather to optimize it if the patient does not use the resource adequately. In any case, individual attention will be given after the session to those patients who require it (e.g., to help someone learn to use the Microsoft Outlook diary or the reminder notes on a mobile phone). Take into account that the different types of external aid can be combined: e.g., add a post-it with the shopping list in the diary the day we go shopping.

As a warm-up exercise, before the new session we do two rounds (one in each direction) working on mental calculation. For example, in the first round we start at the number 53 and each person adds 5, and in the second round we start at 100 and each subtracts 3.

We start by talking about the diary and the different formats available (traditional paper or electronic version).

Patients who do not have a diary are encouraged to buy one for the following session. A very useful type of diary may be one that allows planning of the activities of the day on the left-hand side (prospective memory), while on the right-hand side other information can be written in a notebook-like format. This can also include notes related to therapeutic compliance, mood state, and the hours of sleep, a relevant personal event (e.g., enjoying a day in the spa) or national or international news that has had a particular impact (e.g., the day of the earthquake or tsunami in Japan in 2011).

We try to de-stigmatize the use of the diary to promote its use, since it will improve patient independence and involve mental effort, which may help to increase the ability to encode and retrieve information. Explain the important points to take into account with respect to the use of the work diary:

■ It is important to create a habit of establishing a time in the morning to know the activities of the day.

■ Create a habit at the end of the day of checking what has and has not been done, in order to plan the following day(s); the activities not accomplished during the day will be proposed for the following day or whenever possible (realistic expectations).

■ Always carry the diary in order to note down what should be done at any time; if it is not carried, note the activity down on arrival home.

■ It is important to be specific when noting the tasks (e.g., "go to the supermarket" is not specific enough; we should write "buy bread, eggs, and flour").

After this session, brief individual interviews (5–10 minutes) will be conducted at the end of each session, to revise correct use of the diary.

It is important for the diary used to be manageable and appropriate to the needs of the user. Whatever system is preferred, based on the needs of each patient, we try to promote establishing routines by using only one system rather than several, which could cause confusion. During the following sessions, the therapists should ensure that the chosen procedure is being used efficiently, and this may require some brief appointments with the patients after the sessions. These appointments are useful in case of individual doubts about the use or implementation of the different techniques.

Homework

■ The main task of this session is that of starting to become familiar with the use of the diary.

■ Some mental calculation exercises may be proposed, as well as exercises involving searching for hidden words in a puzzle format and searching for differences between two texts.

Diary

■ Autonomy.

■ Enhance independence.

■ The use of these strategies involves mental effort that can help to increase the ability to encode and retrieve information.

■ It is very important to have the diary at hand when we need to note something down.

■ Check it every day at the same time to check the activities we have and have not done.

■ Plan the next day.

■ When we note down tasks it is important to be specific (e.g., "go to the store" is not very specific: we should write "buy bread, eggs, and flour").

Session 7 slide 8

Material for the patient

External aids are objects that any person, with or without memory problems, may use in his or her daily life. These aids have quite a number of advantages, because the training is simpler than for other memory strategies and, in addition, they are also an effective aid to remembering the need to perform actions in the future (prospective memory). For these strategies to be really useful, it is necessary to train with a professional. This is the main objective of this session.

External strategies

■ The use of a diary may help us to remember the things we have to do and that we have already done. Many people use a *personal diary* to help them remember things, even if they have no memory problems.

■ Make *lists* of the tasks we have to do.

■ Write *post-its* at home and stick them in visible places (e.g., on a mirror) to remind ourselves about a specific activity – for example, taking medication at night, calling the dentist, or buying batteries.

■ Ask someone we trust to remind us to do something important on a specific occasion, but not as a general rule.

■ *Alarms* are useful to remind us that we have left some food cooking in the kitchen, for taking medication, or for remembering a meeting, a date, a medical appointment, a birthday, etc. In these cases it is useful to use the mobile phone organizer with an alarm to remind us beforehand that we have something important to do.

■ We can also use *symbolic reminders*, such as moving a ring from one hand to the other, or changing the clock, in order to remember something specific.

■ *Diary*. If you are going to use a diary as a central element in your memory strategy, also note small activities such as buying bread in the diary, and do not forget to review it every day, even if you think you do not have an important appointment scheduled.

Use your imagination to invent a new external ally for your memory, which we can discuss in the group so that the other members can benefit from this strategy or trick.

In this session we will place special emphasis on how to optimize the use of a diary. Using a diary is the principal strategy to compensate for difficulties in recalling information. In general, a diary may be useful for people who experience problems in retaining information related to appointments, plans, or future activities or important dates to remember. For the diary to be really useful it should allow rapid access to the information and the development of an easy notation system.

The diary may also be used as a notebook, since it may contain different sections responding to different needs.

Data that it may contain:

■ Orientation: data that may orient us at a personal, temporal, and/or spatial level. Note some event or important news that has happened that day, either at a personal level or which has an impact on us.

■ Tasks, appointments, activities to be done during the day. You can even note down the steps to take to do these tasks.

■ Shopping list. The specificity of the task is important – e.g., "go to the shop" is not very specific; in this case it would be better to write "buy bread and eggs."

■ Calendar: a section in which the day that has gone by is crossed out, thereby contributing to temporal orientation.

■ Birthdays of relatives and friends: a section in which we can note down the people we should congratulate.

■ Control of therapeutic compliance. Tick off whether we have taken the medication that day or not.

■ Simple registry of our mood state (1 would mean very depressed and 10 very euphoric) and hours of sleep.

For training in the use of the diary, it is important to always note down the most important appointments and activities of the day, even if we think we will remember.

It is important to *create a habit* and *set a time in the morning* to review what is written in the diary, even if we think that nothing has been written. We should take the diary with us to note down what is necessary at the same time. This task should not be left for later because it will be easy to forget. If we do not have it with us one day, it is important to note down the information on arrival home.

It is important to check that everything has been done at the end of the day and plan the next day.

Electronic diaries may be an interesting alternative for people used to working with information technology. Microsoft Office includes a diary in Outlook (the email program), which is composed of a calendar, contacts, tasks, and notes.

Computers and electronic diaries also offer an alarm function that notifies us if there is any important event or appointment, to remind us of a task to be done, or to indicate that we should consult the diary.

In addition to the diary there are other techniques that can be considered as external aids:

■ *Mobile phones* commonly have an option to set a notification, which may be of great help. They are simple to program and serve as a useful reminder. When a notification is created, the message includes the date and time at which the alarm should sound – for example, 03/08/13 at 12:00 with the message "Helen's birthday. Congratulate her."

■ *Post-its* are colored notes with a self-adhesive system that may be placed in visible sites and may be useful for remembering specific isolated facts. It is important to write the date and throw them away once the activity has been performed. For example, stick a post-it on the telephone saying "call John" or "call for a dental appointment." Another post-it on the bathroom mirror might say "take the medication."

■ *Alarms* may be used when we have to do something not immediately but a short time in the future – for example, if we want to take the cake out of the oven after one hour, or call our child's school in two hours' time.

■ *Pill boxes* can be used to organize the different doses of pills through the day, to avoid forgetting them.

Key points
■ Use the diary daily.

■ Use the mobile phone organizer or the computer with notifications and alarms.

■ Use post-its, pill boxes, and other external aids.

Session 8. Internal strategies to improve memory
Objective

In session 7 we tried to potentiate better use of strategies based on external aids. In session 8 patients are for the first time shown some mnemonic rules to carry out a better process of information encoding, to help in the retrieval of this information. The practice is promoted through different tasks during the session, with the objective of later applying the tasks in their daily routine. We can refer to these techniques as *internal strategies*, since it is the patients themselves who should put these tricks or techniques into practice, to learn to adequately organize new information so that access to this information is more effective. This group of techniques promotes a more profound processing, elaborating the information so that it acquires a structure with more significance. The main techniques to be specifically explained are *association*, *categorization*, and *narration* or story-telling technique.

Session procedure/guidelines for the therapist

Collect the task the patients were assigned in the previous session, briefly discussing it for around 10 minutes.

Prior to the session, we do two warm-up rounds (one in each direction) to work on mental arithmetic. For example, in the first round each person adds 6, starting from number 43, and in the second round they each subtract 4, starting from the number 90.

We start the session with a more theoretical part, explaining some internal strategies that may be used, such as grouping or chunking the information for better organization and remembering. Another possible example would be to establish the habitual use of a specific place for objects at home (e.g., for keys, glasses, handbag, wallet).

Thereafter the **association** technique is explained to the patients. This consists in linking new information with something already known, that is, connecting or linking one element with another. After explaining what the technique consists of, we propose an exercise involving associating pairs of words to remember, firstly in order. We read the list aloud while showing the slide for one minute. Then we ask for the word that matches each of the words. This is an individual task. On completion of the exercise the possible mistakes and strategies used are discussed. Strategies for creating mental images for making associations are provided. We then show the slide again for 30 seconds, after which we again ask for the matching words, but this time out of sequence.

1. Association exercises

- Association is another important element in the development of memory. To associate means simply to connect, join, or link one element with another.

- The association technique is for linking new information to something already known.

Another technique that is worked on is **categorization**, which helps to organize information. This consists in grouping information into categories, thus making sense of the data and facilitating information storage. Several exercises related to this technique are performed, based on organizing words into categories, progressively increasing in complexity. In the first exercise a small number of categories is provided. In the second exercise the patients themselves create the categories, and in the third exercise the number of words to be memorized and the number of possible categories is increased. Given the complexity of this last task, it can be done in pairs.

2. Categorization exercises

- Categorization is a technique that helps to organize information and facilitate memory.

- It consists of grouping information into blocks, using a feature that the items have in common.

- Identifying the common features of the data makes sense of the data and facilitates information storage.

Session 8 slide 13

Lastly, we explain the **story-telling** technique, which consists in inventing a simple story related to the information to be recalled, to thereby more easily facilitate memory. After explaining the technique we propose an individual exercise. A series of words is given on a slide. The patients are asked to write a story using the "target" words. Next, the homework is described, as a distraction. Finally, we ask the patients to write the words used in the story again.

3. Narrative exercises

■ Invent a story about the information that has to be stored. This is an excellent technique to make information easier to remember.

■ Example: "Invent a story containing the words: red, woman, skirt, hill, different, fresh, and neighbors."

Session 8 slide 14

Homework

To continue practicing the internal strategies explained during the session, we propose two exercises as homework:

■ Prepare a shopping list for next week.

■ List the criteria that they would follow to pack a suitcase for a one-week beach holiday.

Material for the patient

In the previous two sessions we started to talk about memory, the problems associated with memory impairments, and why these difficulties may be present in people with bipolar disorder. Remember that oversights or memory failures are also frequent in the rest of the population, and that these are often associated with age. In the previous session we focused mainly on external aids for improving memory problems. In today's session and the next we will mainly work on internal strategies to improve the storage and recall of information. At the end of the session we will attempt to summarize the useful strategies and proposals or tricks which the group may have to improve some of the problems related to memory.

Internal strategies
Most people have the ability to remember very brief information, such as a telephone number or some of the articles on a specific list. For this we could use the strategy of *chunking* or dividing into small parts. For example, the number of our driver's license, 3286754575, could be more easily remembered as 328 – 6754 – 575. If we have a shopping list, it can be divided into small lists based on groupings such as fruit, cold meats, fish, tinned food, etc. If we make small groups of the things on the list (grouping) we can *organize and remember the information better*. If we have groups classified into categories, we could even find the thing we want more easily in the supermarket and would not have to go up and down the aisles as often.

Normally things are remembered better if they are of specific interest to us, and thus it is important to make information interesting or attractive for ourselves.

It is important to *organize the objects at home well*. If we can establish a set place to put medications, important telephone numbers, documents, tools, keys, handbag, and glasses, we will most certainly have less work and less frustration when searching for them. It is useful to associate the places in which we put these objects with their use: the briefcase should be under the desk, the drugs one has to take together with the food in the kitchen, the keys to home on a tray near the door, etc.

More associations. In relation to what we have mentioned up to now, our brain often thinks in images, and it is therefore important to use our imagination to create mental images to thereby retain the necessary information more easily. We will continue working on these tricks in the next session.

Key points

■ Associate: for example, creating mental images.

■ Categorize: for example, using shopping lists.

■ Invent stories including the information that has to be stored.

■ Establish a set place to put medications, important telephone numbers, documents, tools, keys, handbag, glasses, etc.

Session 9. Other mnemonic strategies and their application in daily life

Objective

In this session we continue working on the use of mnemonic techniques that may be useful in the daily life of the patients. We aim to provide a number of different techniques, from among which the patients can choose those which they feel most comfortable with and which they consider to be of greatest utility, potentiating their strong points. That is, our intention is not to practice all of the techniques but rather for the patients to have a range of possibilities.

In this session we again insist that using these techniques may initially require greater effort, but will increasingly improve after the patient has practiced them a number of times. Memory techniques help to make sense of information that previously made no sense, by means of organizing, associating, or making mental images.

Session procedure/guidelines for the therapist

Following the usual methodology, we start by collecting the task that the patients were assigned in the previous session and briefly discuss it for around 10 minutes.

Afterwards we do two warm-up rounds (one in each direction) to work on mental arithmetic. In the first round we start at the number 55 and each person adds 4, and in the second round we start at 100 and each person subtracts 6.

People with bipolar disorder often complain of problems in remembering the names of people. We therefore start by providing some techniques to try to improve remembering names.

How to remember personal names

- ▪ To remember the names of people it is important to:
  - ❑ Pay attention to the name of a person that you have to remember.
  - ❑ Repeat the name several times during the conversation.
  - ❑ Associate the name with that of another person you already know, or create a mental image linking the name and the person (e.g. Elizabeth with a crown – Queen Elizabeth).
  - ❑ Associate some trait characterizing the person and associate it with the name. For example, "Tom is tall" (tall starts with the letter "T" like his name).

- ▪ We can do an exercise with the members of the group if the names are not yet well learned.

Session 9 slide 2

To consolidate this technique we do an exercise to work on the association of names with faces. A slide with photographs of faces and the respective names is shown for two minutes. Then the same faces are shown, in a different order, with no names, and the patients have to give the name corresponding to each face. Once this exercise has been completed we give, as an example, some possible cues for associating the names with some concept to facilitate remembering. For example: John–Jolly, Gareth–Good person, Sandra–Smile, Hannah–Happy, Laura–Lips, Gary–Gorgeous. They can also associate these new names with people they know with the same name.

Another frequent complaint among these patients is the loss of or the inability to find everyday objects. We explain the restitution technique to find lost objects.

Some memory techniques

- **Rhythm** and **rhyme.**

- **Regrouping** information: pairs and acronyms.

- Make **associations** between elements to remember by constructing **mental images.**

- **Repetition** technique.

- **Method of loci**. Make an imaginary journey through a building, putting an idea or image in each room or office. You can retrieve ideas/information by following a virtual tour through the rooms of the building.

Session 9 slide 7

After explaining these techniques we briefly introduce other possible memory strategies, such as rhythm and rhyme, regrouping (acronyms), repetition, and the method of loci.

We explain the method of loci in greater detail. This method consists in making an imaginary route through a building such as the person's home, or along a usual pathway, placing an idea or image in each room or at each specific place. After creating these associations we can retrieve the ideas by following a virtual route through the places where the ideas were left. The technique is based on creating a map or mental pathway that is used, together with visual images, as a tool to remember a series of items or elements that we wish to memorize in the correct order. After explaining this technique and giving an example to facilitate comprehension, we put it into practice with an exercise. For example, the group is asked to remember a list of objects based on this method, with each person making a mental pathway through five rooms of his or her house. After doing a distracting task they should recall the list they have memorized. This technique requires a lot of practice to do well, but can be very effective.

Afterwards, we begin to work on verbal memory. We read some news aloud, or play some previously recorded news as if we were listening to the radio. Once the group has listened to the news, we show some questions on the screen, for them to answer individually on a sheet of paper. The questions are given one by one, with a maximum of approximately 30 seconds to answer each question. Afterwards the answers will be discussed in small groups. After all the questions have been answered, the news is shown in written form on a slide, so that the answers can be checked.

Another type of exercise that can be carried out is to give an illustration of a travel agency advertisement, for instance. The group is asked to read it carefully. After approximately one minute a version of the slide is shown with some of the text blanked out, and the missing information should be filled in with the information they remember. Once this has been done, the information will be compared with the original. This exercise can be explained using the technique of vanishing cues, which is another useful way to learn short pieces of verbal information that you want to keep in mind, for example addresses.

Lastly, the homework to be done is explained, and a volunteer is asked to read the key points of the session aloud.

Homework

■ Memorize a short poem by a well-known author, or the verse of a chosen song.

■ Describe the criteria to be followed in organizing kitchen and bathroom cabinets so as to easily find a specific utensil or product. In any case it will be easier to remember where it is located if a space is orderly or organized.

■ Optional exercise: the patients carefully read a text, and then are shown the same text with some words missing, in which they must fill in the blanks from memory.

Material for the patient

In this session we will review the internal strategies covered in the previous session and continue practicing new mnemonic strategies.

We will reinforce the association exercises, linking the new information with something we already know. We will also work in more depth on the categorization exercises. This technique will help us to organize the information based on one of our senses and thereby facilitate subsequent storage in memory.

We will propose new exercises based on relationships, that is, inventing stories about the information (words) we wish to memorize. It is easier to remember concepts when we find a relationship between them.

Another common complaint of patients is a difficulty in remembering the names of new people. To **remember names** it is important to pay attention to the name of the person you wish to remember, repeat the name several times during the conversation, associate the name with another known name, or associate a feature that characterizes the person with the name. For example: "Tom is tall" – where *tall* starts with the letter T, like his name. It may also be useful to associate the name with that of someone famous, or a relative.

One of the situations that makes us uncomfortable is **losing an object** or not remembering where we have put it. First of all we should look in areas of the house where we normally leave this object, even if we do not remember having left it there. Then we should go over the places where we forgot it the last time, and lastly we should review the unusual activities we have done during the day to see if this gives us some indication.

Other memorization techniques that also give some information and that may be useful for associating, organizing, and creating mental images are **rhythm and rhyming** and **acronyms**.

Through rhythm and rhyme we can repeat specific data that we want to remember over and over again, following the rhythm of a song or making a rhyme, promoting memory rather than comprehension in this case. This happens, for example, when we memorize the multiplication tables. We will memorize poems by known authors and the verse of a chosen song following this strategy.

If we wish to remember important issues related to bipolar disorder we could use the acronym DEMSAT (early DE, detection; M, medication; S, sleep; A, accept disease; T, toxic substances).

The **repetition** technique consists of mentally repeating the information we wish to retain. In this way we force ourselves to focus on this information, increasing the possibility of memorizing it. This may be useful when going from one room to another at home with the intention of doing something, and we mentally repeat what we want to do to avoid any interference en route.

Key points

■ If we organize the information it will be easier to remember it.

■ Convert the new information which we have to remember into an image or data kept in our memory. We can also help ourselves with verbal associations such as rhymes.

Session 10. Reading and remembering

Objective

Some patients complain about not remembering the novels they have read, and even forget the title and/or the name of the author. This can be discouraging and frustrating, and can even make them abandon the reading habit.

The long-term objective of this session is get patients to reacquire the reading habit, in the case that they have lost it, or to acquire the habit in those who do not have it. With this objective in mind, we give a series of guidelines during the session, while proposing the reading of a book to be discussed in each session through questions formulated within the context of the homework.

Session procedure/guidelines for the therapist

At the beginning of the session we ask about the participants' week and whether there are any questions about the previous session. Then we ask if a volunteer would like to recite a verse from a poem or song that they have learned during the week.

Next we do two warm-up rounds (one in each direction) to work on mental arithmetic, starting at 22 and adding 9 each time, and then starting at 85 and subtracting 3.

Before starting on the new content we review sessions 6, 7, 8, and 9, which were devoted to external and internal memory strategies, to ensure that they are clear and to assess whether they are being used.

Mnemonic strategies: summary

External strategies

- Diary
- Personal journal
- Lists of things and "to do's" (group/divide)
- Post-its
- Ask a trusted person to remember an appointment
- Alarms
- Mobile organizer
- Symbolic reminder (e.g., change watch or ring)
- Pill-box
- Calendar

Session 10 slide 2

Internal strategies

- Story-telling technique (the shorter the better): using verbal mediators to make mental associations
- Split or "chunk" the information (e.g., pairs)
- Association (e.g., dog – car: the dog is in the car)
- Categorization (e.g., shopping lists, packing a suitcase, ...)
- Rhythm, rhyme: they do not ensure understanding but do help remembering (e.g., multiplication tables)
- Acronyms – e.g., IODOCO (Ionic, Doric, Corinthian)
- Repetition technique
- Method of loci: a picture or mental association with a particular place

Session 10 slide 3

We begin the new content with a general, very simple guideline on reading: start reading in "doses." It is not necessary to read for one hour continuously; it is better to break it up into shorter sessions – e.g., 15 minutes before eating, 10 minutes in the afternoon, 20 minutes after dinner.

Then we propose other guidelines based on whether what is being read is a newspaper article or a novel:

- For a news article, three steps should be followed: (1) start with a general reading, without noting down anything, but attempting to relate the content to information that is already known; (2) recite the most important points (ask yourself *who*, *what*, *when*, *where*, *why*, and *how*), since news usually responds to these questions; (3) mentally review what has just been read, to consolidate the fundamental ideas.

- For a novel, it is recommended that patients should start by reading a simple novel, and that they should use a notebook to write down relevant information: (1) the date they started reading the book and when it was finished; (2) the title and author(s); (3) a brief summary of each chapter or an overall synthesis; (4) finally, a personal opinion, since memories associated with emotional memory are more easily retrieved than those that have not triggered any emotion.

We do two tasks during the session. Firstly, a text of approximately 150 words is handed out to all the members of the group. They will be given four minutes to read it. As a guideline, they are advised to underline the ideas or information they consider important in the text. Then *in pairs* they should respond to the previously prepared questions, for which they are given a further four minutes without the text in front of them.

The next task is also based on reading a text. They are again given four minutes to read it, but in this case the questions are answered individually. Then we put the answers to the two texts together.

Finally, to finish the session, we encourage a volunteer to read the key points of the session aloud.

Homework

To facilitate the recovery or reacquisition of the reading habit we propose reading the book *The Little Prince* by Antoine de Saint-Exupéry. Starting with this session and until the end of the program we propose that three chapters be read each week, using the method explained during the session. The patients will also have to answer a series of questions on each chapter, to enable them to better assimilate the content of the book. As to the choice of the book, it should be said that *The Little Prince* is only our proposal. If you think that the content of this book is too symbolic for the level of your group, or if you simply prefer to work with another format (e.g., short stories), that is possible. You will have to adapt the questions to the book chosen. The objective is to have follow-up work at home on the reading of a book or texts.

■ For the next session they will have to have read the first three chapters of the book and answer the questions (see *Questions and answers on The Little Prince*, in the online material for the therapist).

■ Another task will be to choose a current news article on an issue of interest and follow that issue in the news until the end of the group sessions. Alternatively, news on a different topic can be chosen each week.

■ Memorize a new verse of the poem started in the previous session.

Material for the patient

We often have the sensation that shortly after finishing a book we remember practically nothing about what we have read. This may be a very general impression, but sometimes it may even be difficult to remember the title or author of the book. This is, on occasions, very discouraging, particularly in the case of patients who were avid readers and who, over time, and especially during depressive episodes, have experienced difficulties in concentration. In addition, after the episodes of the disease, it is difficult for some people with bipolar disorder to recover the reading habit. Many patients mention that they continue to have problems concentrating, and many others do not remember what they are reading.

Provided that the patient is not in the middle of an acute episode, we recommend that reading be attempted, although not for prolonged periods of time. In the case of physical exercise, it is not necessary to run for two hours; it is sufficient to walk quickly for 10 minutes first thing in the morning, 15 minutes before lunch, and another 15 minutes afterwards, and 15 or 20 minutes in the afternoon. This would make up an hour of physical exercise (although not all at once) per day. We can do the same with reading: when we attempt to generate or recover a **habit**, we can **implement it little by little**, even though it is difficult to maintain our attention for a long time. In this way, we can maintain our attention focused for progressively longer periods of time.

It is better to start with a simple text or a newspaper or magazine article, rather than first choosing *Pride and Prejudice* or *Crime and Punishment*, for example.

If we read an **article** in the newspaper we can follow the three-steps strategy known as **3R (read, recite, and review)**, in order to improve our retention of the most important information. The steps are as follows:

1st   Start with a general **reading** without highlighting or taking notes.

2nd   Next, **recite** what is most important (it may be useful to answer the six questions that form the basis of good journalism: *who, what, when, where, why,* and *how*).

3rd   Mentally **review** the most relevant information you have just read.

For those interested in more complex texts, such as students and those who have to read books or chapters, it may be useful to follow the **SQ3R** reading method (survey, question, read, recite, and review). This method is similar to others such as the PQRST strategy, and its practice increases comprehension and retention of information through enhancing organization and data processing:

- **S (survey or skim)**. Make a general overview of the material with the objective of discovering the main topic. In the case of a book, it is important to glance at the chapter title, headings, graphs, the introduction, bold print, etc. Thus, in a few minutes we will gain a better idea of how the information is presented and organized. Also, rapid reading of the summary, if any, may be useful to identify the most relevant data.

- **Q (questions)**. Before we begin reading a section, we should turn the heading into a question. This will increase our active involvement and comprehension, and should also bring to mind information we already know concerning the main topic. The questions we ask ourselves may help make relevant points stand out as we read. If applied, this step forces us to maintain attention and helps to make sense of the information we are working with.

- **3R (read, recite, and review)**. Careful reading of the material to answer the key questions:

(1) **Read** the whole chapter without underlining or taking notes.

(2) Identify and highlight the main ideas, but only after reading a section or once a chapter is finished. Look for answers to the previous questions, establishing associations and relating the information. It may be useful to jot down brief notes. Read and try to mentally **recite** in your own words what the reading is about. This reading is where the most time is spent, and it allows us to check that we have understood the material.

(3) The last reading should be to **review**. This helps us to maintain and consolidate the main ideas. Check your memory by reciting the main points out loud, making sure you understand them.

On most occasions we will be reading a novel. It is recommended to start with a simple novel, or short stories, or poems. A good system to remember what we have read may be to have a *notebook* or a file to collect relevant information:

- The date on which the book was started and when it was finished.

- The title and author(s).

- A brief summary of each chapter and/or a final synthesis.

- Including at the end our opinion or personal impression. The opinion we have of the book we have read will help us remember the general argument better, since it implies a more in-depth elaboration of the material read.

Key points

- Use the guidelines for reading news: reviewing the material, then reciting the most important data, and finally making a mental review of the most relevant information.

- Attempt to relate the new information to what you already know (for example, when you follow a news report).

- Generate an opinion with respect to what you have read, to help retain the information.

Session 11. Puzzles: retrieving information from the past
Objective

Many patients complain of an inability to remember important parts of their lives. This situation produces sadness, a sense of impotence, and often a conflict with their relatives who do not understand how they cannot remember such an important date or event for the family. In this session we work on some strategies that allow the reconstruction of this information from the past.

Session procedure/guidelines for the therapist

Collect the tasks from the previous session and discuss them for approximately 10 minutes.

We start with two rounds of mental arithmetic, one in each direction. In the first round they add 9, starting with the number 22, and in the second round they subtract 3, starting from 85.

We then start with the content of the new session. We suggest material which will support the storing of memories, such as a personal diary, a recorder, photographs, a video camera, or the help of relatives or close friends.

As work to be done during the session we propose that they think about some significant event in their lives. This exercise is done in pairs. Each of the two partners in turn explains an event, and the other asks questions to clarify the information. Afterwards, each member of a pair briefly summarizes what their partner has explained.

To work on aspects of semantic memory we show the photographs of 35 well-known people from different settings. Each image is shown for about 15 seconds. A patient who does not remember the name of the person is asked to identify the professional field for which the person is known. The patients have to recognize the persons individually and afterwards discuss the identity of the people in small groups of four or five patients.

Homework

- Collect information on a recent trip or outing (look at photos at home, remember the route followed, the places visited, etc.).

- Write down a selection of titles of songs which are of significance to you, adding the name of the singers or groups if you remember them.

- Make a list of movies you have seen, with the names of the stars and, if you remember, when you saw each one.

- Continue reading the book and answer the questions (see *Questions and answers on The Little Prince*, in the online material for the therapist).

- Summarize the news relating to the issue you have chosen to follow.

Material for the patient

We often have the impression that our autobiography is incomplete, and that we are missing data from the past. This may be due, in part, to the episodes of the disease, which sometimes represent a break in our personal life story. During the episodes of mania and depression, our thoughts, emotions, and behavior are different from usual and may even lead to hospitalization because of their severity. This represents a disruption in the functioning of the patient, and patients mention that they have forgotten part of what happened during the episodes, especially during manic episodes.

Some patients have the perception that they remember their lives as fragmented by the interruptions due to relapses, while others report difficulty in chronologically ordering important events in their lives.

This is why it is important to use strategies to reconstruct information from the past, and, for the future, to be able to retrieve information that may be relevant in our lives.

In session 7, we commented that it would be interesting to use a **diary** as a tool to make brief notes of personal events which are significant, and thereby to have a record of those events.

Additionally, many people, whether or not they have bipolar disorder, use a **personal diary** to note those day-to-day situations or experiences that they wish to keep a record of, because it is impossible to remember everything, as we discussed in the first sessions.

Other tools that may be useful instead of a diary would be to use a **recorder** with the same function as a diary, keeping a register of the everyday events or experiences which we wish to record or remember. For special occasions (birthdays, weddings, Christmas, parties, trips, etc.), it might be useful to take **photographs** or use a **video camera** following a certain order, specifying some data (date, place, who was there, funny anecdotes, etc.) in the photo album or explained in the video or DVD.

Using the metaphor of our brain as a computer, all these tools (diary, recorder, notebook, camera, or video) would be like a type of external hard disk to which we can enter information for later retrieval. To facilitate access to the information stored, it is recommended to organize the diaries, notebooks, or videos using clear labels (e.g., in the videos or DVDs specify the date or the event recorded – for example, "Helen's christening" – or in the case of a diary you could note the period or year).

It may sometimes be necessary to retrieve information from our past, to reconstruct the different pieces as if they were a puzzle, attempting to put them into their place with the **help of a relative or close friends** who may provide the necessary information (through data which they may provide us such as photographs, videos, letters, or emails). In this way we will be able to access the memory of some vacation or other special dates.

In addition to the information making up our autobiography, during our lifetime we incorporate knowledge corresponding to semantic memory, which we mentioned previously in session 6. This knowledge includes historical events, films we have seen, books we have read, writers, musicians, politicians, etc. It is important to activate this information, since if it is not correctly saved following some order or criterion, it will be more difficult to retrieve (recall the metaphor of memory as a library, from session 6). In this and the following sessions we will do some tasks to stimulate or activate these data which are stored and which are sometimes difficult to retrieve.

Key points

■ The diary may be a crucial aid, to be consulted, albeit briefly, when we need to recall situations or significant personal experiences. In addition, we have the advantage of having the information organized by years. In a personal diary this information may be more fully described.

■ The organization of memories using photographs that are well classified and recordings or videos of important events that are adequately labeled will facilitate the retrieval of information from our past.

Module 4. Executive functions

We begin a new block of five sessions in which we work on aspects related to the executive functions. As explained in the first introductory sessions, the executive functions include a group of functions that are usually related mainly to the frontal lobes, and that allow us to organize, plan, and direct our behavior towards a specific goal and give us the ability to carry it out efficiently. Thus, these functions allow us to constantly adapt to the changes required by the environment around us. It should be taken into account that many of the cognitive complaints experienced by patients with bipolar disorder are related more to the executive functions than, for example, to true deficits in memory or attention. The main problem is that patients are not aware of these difficulties, or that they do not recognize them as part of their cognitive deficits. This module is about training in executive functions, giving the patients guidelines to help with organizing, planning, solving problems, establishing priorities, and time management, taking into account self-instructions and other strategies.

Session 12. Executive functions: self-instructions and self-monitoring
Objective

In this session we focus on the planning, implementation, and monitoring of activities aimed at an objective.

Session procedure/guidelines for the therapist

Before starting the session we should take into account that we will need material including maps of our city and public transportation (for example, the metro and buses) to do some of the practical tasks.

Briefly discuss the task from the previous session (approximately 10 minutes).

We do two warm-up rounds to work on verbal fluency. For example, in the first round the patients have to say words beginning with the letter T, and in the second round they should give words beginning with the letter C.

We begin the theoretical part of the session by explaining the main executive functions and the main clinical manifestations of problems with them, such as difficulties in planning activities or in retrieving words, getting lost in new situations, etc.

The executive functions

The main executive functions can be summarized as three:

- **Planning**: deciding on the best course of action.
- **Implementation**: putting the plan decided upon into practice.
- **Monitoring**: closely following the plan to see if it is effective and, if not, making the necessary changes.

Problems in these areas can significantly affect a patient's occupational, interpersonal, and social functioning.

Session 12 slide 2

How are disturbances in the executive functions manifested ?

- ❑ Difficulty in organizing tasks in an orderly way
- ❑ Easily distracted
- ❑ Difficulty in problem solving
- ❑ Difficulty in planning activities
- ❑ Slow in making changes in routine
- ❑ Difficulty in retrieving words, "tip of tongue"
- ❑ Feeling lost in new situations
- ❑ Difficulty in doing long routine tasks

Session 12 slide 3

It should be taken into account that the patients usually have great lack of knowledge regarding executive functions. Although the concept has been introduced in the first few sessions, many of the patients do not precisely remember what we are referring to when we talk about executive functions. We take the necessary time to ensure that the concept is clear to all.

Afterwards, we focus on the *steps necessary to carry out and complete an activity aimed at a specific goal*: (1) know the steps that need to be followed to complete the activity, (2) establish the sequence of the steps, (3) launch the plan, and (4) review the plan and introduce modification in the case of unforeseen events. In addition, we provide some guidelines that may facilitate this sequence. One of the key metacognitive strategies is the use of self-instructions and even material such as diagrams, lists, notes, etc., which facilitate or guide the behavior to follow and the sequence of steps to follow.

Guidelines

- ❏ Stop and think about what we need to do.
- ❏ Define the main task to be performed.
- ❏ Record each of the necessary steps to accomplish a particular task.
- ❏ Over time you can learn the steps without writing them down, automate the process (e.g., a recipe).
- ❏ Check that you are following the steps while performing the task.

Session 12 slide 5

Next, we do an activity in pairs to demonstrate the utility of establishing a predetermined order to correctly perform a task with a specific aim. For example, the patients could work out the steps to be taken, and the order to follow, to make a Spanish omelette.

Next, we focus on *time management*, that is, the ability to adequately judge the time necessary to perform different activities and regulate the behavior according to the time restriction. Again, we provide a series of guidelines for the patients, to facilitate learning to manage their time with greater efficacy when programming and planning activities.

Guidelines

- Grade the complexity of the tasks.
- Simple, clear self-instructions that help to structure and execute the task.
- Encourage the use of internal strategies for specific situations, such as impulse control (e.g., self-instruction as in "think before you act" or "go slowly").
- Plan tasks ahead, and be realistic about what we can do in a given period of time.

Session 12 slide 8

Following the practical work, we do some more tasks in situ. Among these, we first propose the planning and performance of routes in our own city (for example, "going from my house to the zoo and from the zoo to the opera on the metro"). In these tasks it would be convenient to provide a map of the metro and another of the city. This should be adapted to the city where the center is based. In the case of the metro, patients should note down the different changes in line necessary and, if walking, the streets that they will follow. Moreover, patients have to estimate the time needed to get from one place to another. This task should take approximately five minutes, and they can work in pairs.

Then we explain the steps of a story out of order and, working individually, they have to put the story into a logical order. The same type of exercise can be done with phrases from a conversation, which we can invent.

Another optional activity (depending on the time available) consists of proposing a series of activites in which the patients should list all the steps that need to be followed, in the correct order – to look for a flat to rent, for example, or to join a gymnasium, etc. Other alternatives can be substituted, if these tasks are too complicated.

Lastly, we explain the homework and ask a volunteer to read out the key points.

Homework

- Look at the clock when you believe that two minutes or a quarter of an hour has passed (this task can be done with or without distractors).
- Within a natural setting, estimate how long it would take to go from your house to the hospital, from your house to the supermarket, etc., and then check this.
- Organize a one-day tour for a friend. Imagine that next Saturday an old friend of yours is coming to visit. He or she has never been to your city, so you will have to be the tourist guide for the whole day. Help yourself with the following guidelines:

(1)   Your friend will arrive at the train station at 8 a.m. What do you do first?

(2)   Describe the route you have planned for the morning, with the sights you consider interesting to visit (you must take account of the time necessary in each place and the time it takes to get there).

(3)   Think about a place to go for lunch (consider typical dishes that you would recommend that your friend should try).

(4)   After a short rest you will continue with the tour. Where will you take your friend?

(5)   Your friend wants to buy a souvenir of the city for a relative. What would you recommend? Where can you find it?

■ Continue working on the news chosen in the previous session. If that is not possible, choose another news article of interest.

■ Read chapters 7, 8, and 9 of *The Little Prince* and answer the questions (see *Questions and answers on The Little Prince*, in the online material for the therapist).

■ Optional exercise: organize an activity such as a weekend outing, taking into account the following points:

(1)   In what order would you do the tasks, and why have you chosen this order?

(2)   Estimate the time needed to carry out each of the tasks.

(3)   Introduce changes requiring an adjustment in the activities (e.g., it rains the day of the outing).

Material for the patient

The **executive functions** are defined as a group of cognitive abilities that allow anticipation and the establishment of goals, programming and organization of activities, self-regulation of tasks, and the ability to carry them out efficiently. These functions are linked to the frontal brain lobes. The executive functions act as the "orchestra conductor" of the brain.

According to this metaphor the frontal lobes of the brain are responsible for receiving information from the rest of the cerebral structures and coordinating them to perform behaviors directed towards an objective.

What are executive functions for?

■ They help us perceive what is around us.

■ They help us execute complex actions with an objective.

■ They intervene in the capacity of solving everyday problems at home and at work.

■ They help to direct the attention towards specific information, inhibiting irrelevant stimuli (selective attention), and therefore allow us to fight against involuntary distractions, that is, dispensing with irrelevant information.

■ They allow us to remember priorities, by recognizing hierarchies and the significance of the stimuli we perceive.

■ They allow us to formulate a plan to start or inhibit activities, modify strategies according to the priority of the plan, and maintain a sequence of activities and effort.

■ Flexibility: they enable us to adapt the behavior to environmental changes.

The main executive functions may be summarized as three: planning, implementation, and monitoring.

Bipolar patients may show problems in these areas, but what problems do they have when there are difficulties in the executive functions?

■ Difficulty in the ability to neatly organize tasks.

■ Prone to distraction.

- Difficulty in solving problems.
- Difficulties in the planning of activities.
- Slow in making changes in routine.
- Difficulty in finding words (tip-of-the-tongue experience).
- Feeling lost in new situations.
- Difficulty in large tasks.

On some occasions when a patient complains of memory problems and/or feeling distracted, the problem is not in the memory but rather in the executive functions. Characteristic expressions of people with these difficulties are: "The word is on the tip of my tongue," "Anything can distract me," "I can't organize myself," "I cannot finish what I want to do."

All brain activities require concentration. The information comes quickly and from many places at the same time – someone talking to us, the television, noise from the street – and this reduces the attention, that is, our thoughts disperse and we believe that we used to solve problems more quickly. It becomes difficult to analyze a situation, find a solution, and carry it out. It becomes somewhat more difficult to adapt to new situations or changes in routine. Patients often complain that it is very difficult for them to "organize themselves," even delaying activities they have to do. They also show many difficulties in managing time. They realize that time does not go as far as it should. Many patients taking the morning off may arrive late for an appointment due to lack of anticipation.

The rehabilitation of executive functions constitutes an essential objective of any cognitive rehabilitation or remediation program, since this deficit is responsible for some important obstacles in everyday life.

Some general suggestions are:

(1) Grade the complexity of the tasks from lesser to greater.

(2) Divide the task into several steps or separate components.

(3) Give yourself clear, simple instructions which help to structure and execute the task (order the steps).

(4) Use the most accessible resources (e.g., if we wish to find our way to a new place we can consult a map or telephone to ask how to get there).

(5) Use internal strategies (self-instructions such as "think before acting", "keep calm," "this is the next step").

(6) How long do you need to do this task? We might think, for example, that we need 30 minutes to get from our house to work, but we are only taking the bus route into account. We must also consider that it takes 5 minutes to get to the bus stop and 10 more minutes from the time we get off the bus to reach our workplace.

(7) Think that on some occasions something unexpected might occur, which might compel us to modify the expected order of the activities.

(8) It is fundamental to establish and maintain a personal timetable. Avoid leaving everything to the last minute, since this may increase the level of stress. It is also important to know what is relevant in our life and what is accessory. It is therefore advisable to make a list or plan the tasks we have to do in order of priority.

In this and the following sessions we will see some examples of how to better organize ourselves and give priority to what is the most important or urgent.

Key points

- The executive functions allow us to neatly organize and plan, solve problems, and adapt behavior to environmental changes.

■ It is important to grade the complexity of the tasks, divide the task into several steps, consider how long we need to carry out each task, and give priority to what is most important, taking into account that sometimes something unexpected might occur.

■ If we use self-instructions and are aware of the steps we must take to carry out a task, the end result will be the most effective.

Session 13. Executive functions: programming and organizing activities

Objective

This session is practical, working on the concepts acquired in session 12, such as the planning of activities and time management in the self-regulation of tasks.

Session procedure/guidelines for the therapist

Following the usual methodology, we begin the session by discussing the tasks which were to be done at home during the previous week.

As a warm-up, we do two rounds (one in each direction) to work on verbal fluency. For example, in the first round they might say the names of persons starting with the letter A, and in the second round they might give the names of European cities.

In this session we divide the group into two subgroups. One subgroup of patients works on a planning task outside the classroom, while the other remains inside, doing a similar task with pencil and paper.

The first subgroup goes outside the building to carry out a series of five tasks around the center, taking a maximum of 20 minutes. The patients are not allowed to take a watch, so that they gain practice in making an approximate calculation of the time. Likewise, we will work on issues related to memory functions, since they do not write down the five tasks, but must memorize them. The specific activities to be undertaken can be modified according to the location of the center. It is important to remind them that, despite being in a group, the tasks should be carried out individually. One of the therapists can accompany them for supervision. As an example, the following five tasks might be proposed:

(1)   Make a photocopy of your identity card, or something similar.

(2)   Ask about the price of 1 kg of tomatoes in a nearby shop.

(3)   Buy a small bottle of water.

(4)   Go to the newspaper stand and note down a headline from the *Financial Times* or the *Sun* for that day.

(5)   Look up the opening hours of a shop on the corner.

For the pencil-and-paper exercise to be done by the other subgroup in the classroom, we provide a map of an amusement park with a series of specific places to visit, following some specific rules.

Amusement park

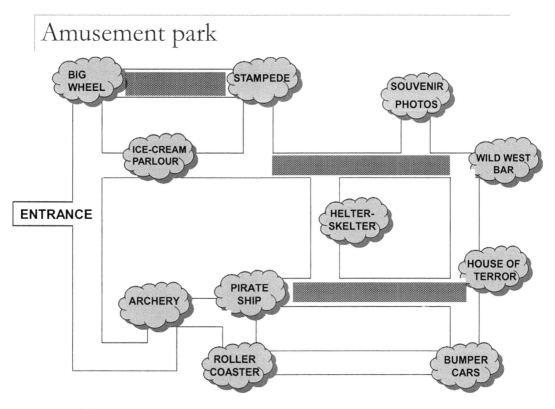

Session 13 slide 3

Rules

- **Places to visit:**
  - Bumper cars, helter-skelter, and stampede (not necessarily in that order).

- **Rules:**
  - Start at the entrance and finish at the souvenir photos.
  - The shaded pathways can only be used **once**.

Session 13 slide 4

As an additional task, an alternative version of this exercise is done, based on the same map, but this time stipulating that the places must be visited in a specified order.

Amusement park: second version

Session 13 slide 6

This exercise should be done individually.

Once the two groups have finished their tasks, they should discuss the difficulties they each encountered, and what alternative procedures they had in each case.

Another practical task which we propose is to describe the steps necessary to prepare for a two-week holiday, for example in India. They can be given approximately 10 minutes to list the steps to prepare for this vacation and then discuss them together.

Lastly, explain the homework.

Homework

■ Organize an activity that is out of the ordinary, such as a birthday party, with the help of the following list:
   (a)   In what order will you do the tasks, and why?
   (b)   Estimate the time needed to carry out each of the tasks.
   (c)   Introduce a change that requires an adjustment in the planning (e.g., someone is allergic to the food prepared).

■ Continue working on the follow-up of the news article. If this is not possible choose another article of interest.

■ Read chapters 10, 11, and 12 of *The Little Prince* and answer the questions (see *Questions and answers on The Little Prince*, in the online material for the therapist).

Material for the patient

This session will be devoted to putting into practice the concepts acquired in the previous session, such as the planning of activities and time management in the self-regulation of tasks.

To start with we propose an exercise which should be carried out over a 15-minute period outside the building (you cannot take a watch with you, so you must calculate the time). The activity consists in performing five tasks around the hospital [adapt to suit the center]:

■ Make a photocopy of your ID card or something similar.

■ Ask about the price of 1 kg of tomatoes in a nearby shop.

■ Buy a small bottle of water.

■ Go to a newspaper stand and write down the main headline from the *Financial Times* or the *Sun*.

■ Find out the opening hours of the handbag shop on the corner.

On completion of all the tasks, return to the center and the other group will go out and do the same activity. It is important to note that even though you go out as a group, you must do the tasks by yourself.

We will also revise some aspects of memory worked on in previous sessions. Therefore, you cannot note down the tasks you must do, but rather you will have to remember them.

Meanwhile, with the group that stays in the room, we will do a similar task but with pencil and paper. When both groups have finished the two tasks, we will discuss the difficulties that have been encountered and other strategies to consider in each case.

Key points
■ Planning the order of the activities we have to carry out, and control of time, are two important aspects of better organizing our daily lives.

Session 14. Executive functions: programming activities, establishing priorities, and time management

Objective

The objective of this session is to continue working on issues related to executive functions. Specifically, in this session we review the essential points to take into account when programming day-to-day activities, and we practice exercises based on the organization and programming of more or less complex tasks, establishing priorities.

Session procedure/guidelines for the therapist

Collect the task the patients had from the previous session and discuss it briefly for approximately 10 minutes.

Before beginning the session, we do two warm-up rounds (one in each direction) to work on verbal fluency. In the first, they have to name kitchen utensils, and in the second they should name objects that can be found in an office.

We review the essential points of good time management: programming everyday activities, taking into account the order in which they should be done, asking why this order was chosen, estimating the time expected to carry out each task, and establishing priorities. In the case of an unforeseen event, changes should be introduced into the usual routine, requiring an adjustment in the sequence of activities. It is important to take short rests and, whenever possible, to delegate responsibilities.

We then explain a hypothetical situation in which Helen has to carry out different activities during the day, some of which are urgent while others are not. The patients are each given a chart on which they should individually note down the tasks that Helen must do, in the order they should be done, the time estimated to do them, and the level of urgency.

Time management exercises

Things to be done	Time required for the activity	Urgency	Order in which it should be done

Urgency level: ** urgent, * not urgent

Session 14 slide 5

As the second part of the exercise we add an unforeseen event to the situation. A new chart is provided, on which they should restructure the day based on this last-minute change. At the end of the exercise we discuss the solutions proposed by each member of the group.

We end the session by explaining the homework to be done, and then suggesting that a volunteer read the key points of the session aloud.

Homework

■ They should plan the activities they have to do over the next week, following the chart and the method explained in today's session.

■ We propose three different situations with a problem to be solved. They must continue to employ strategies to find solutions to situations that might arise in real life.

■ Lastly, we continue working on the reading. They should read three more chapters of the book and answer the questions (see *Questions and answers on The Little Prince*, in the online material for the therapist), and a summary of a news article on the chosen topic should be made.

Material for the patient

This is essentially a practical session. Firstly, we will review the main points to take into account when programming activities.

Training in the executive functions requires a great deal of practice, and we therefore propose the organization of one of your routine days, and afterwards other activities that are less usual, such as organizing a surprise birthday party for a relative.

To program everyday activities we have to consider the order in which they will be done and the reason why we have chosen this order, and we will estimate, with the help of a chart, the time needed to do each task.

Once all the steps have been completed, we will include some unforeseen events that could occur and see how the distribution of the activities may need to be adjusted based on these last-minute changes. With this exercise we aim to work on the planning of tasks and establishing priorities, in addition to the capacity of flexibility in the event of possible changes.

Key points

■ Program everyday activities, taking into account:

  ☐ order of execution;
  ☐ time estimation;
  ☐ adapting to unforeseen events.

■ Establish priorities.

■ Take small rests.

■ Delegate responsibilities.

Session 15. Executive functions: problem-solving techniques

Objective

Little by little we are approaching the end of the intervention. This session is devoted to one of the main metacognitive strategies – problem solving, focusing our interest on improving the ability to make responsible autonomous decisions, weighing the pros and cons of the different possible alternatives in a situation. This is done based on the problem-solving technique of D'Zurilla and Goldfried (1971). We discuss techniques for generating alternatives and assessing the possible consequences that may derive from our decisions, and for avoiding making decisions impulsively, without reflection. Decision making is learned, and thus can be practiced and improved. This and the next session are devoted to practicing problem solving.

Session procedure/guidelines for the therapist

We collect the tasks done at home and discuss them briefly. We focus particularly on discussing the planning tasks of a weekday, asking for a volunteer to explain how they carried out the tasks.

Before beginning the session, we do two warm-up rounds (one in each direction) to continue practicing tasks involving verbal fluency. The first round is based on types of flowers, and the second on the names of people beginning with the letter C.

We then explain what problem solving consists of.

Methods

- Analyze the problem calmly, avoiding solving it impulsively. Take time to recognize the problem and formulate it.

- "Brainstorming".

- Choose the solution with the most advantages and the fewest disadvantages/risks.

- Implement the chosen solution.

Session 15 slide 2

Rational problem-solving skills include:

- Problem orientation: attempting to identify a problem when it occurs.
- Problem definition and formulation.
- Generation of alternatives.
- Decision making.
- Implementing the chosen alternatives and verification; evaluating the efficacy of the effort at problem solving.

In the first two steps the point is to analyze the problem calmly, avoiding impulsive resolution and taking time to recognize the problem and express it in words. The third step has to do with "brainstorming", that is, generating possible solutions without being restrictive; we have to note and consider all the ideas which arise without judging them or rapidly ruling them out, although a priori they may seem somewhat impossible. For each alternative we consider the advantages, disadvantages, and risks, assigning a score of 0 to 10 for each one. Next, we should choose the alternative or combination of two or three alternatives with the highest score, and, finally, implement the plan and verify the result of its application.

Once the theory has been explained, we apply the method to a concrete problem proposed by the therapists. This example will be undertaken as a group, noting the contributions of the patients on the board.

We finish the session by explaining the homework and reading the key points of the session aloud.

Homework

■ Think about a relatively uncomplicated problem to work on following this method in the next session.

■ Continue reading the book and answer the questions (see *Questions and answers on The Little Prince*, in the online material for the therapist), and make another summary of a news article.

Material for the patient

In our daily lives we continually encounter problems that must be solved. The presence of problems creates unease, stress, and negative thoughts such as "I can't do anything," "this has no solution," etc., or we have ambivalent feelings. We do not know what to decide or do, leading to feelings of incapacity and impotence.

Bipolar patients often have difficulties in solving problems, and thus we will devote this session to teaching you a simple method that may be applied in problematic situations you may encounter:

(1) Problem **orientation**. Firstly, it is important to have an idea about the nature of the problem that needs to be solved.

(2) Next, the most important thing is to avoid rushing and impulsiveness as we attempt to solve the problem. We must take some time to **recognize the problem and formulate it** clearly. We must analyze the relevant aspects and the factors influencing their appearance and maintenance. You also know that it is advisable to make decisions, and thus to solve problems, when in a euthymic state, so as to avoid the cognitive distortions that provoke the symptoms which appear during an episode.

(3) As a third step it is important to **generate all the possible solutions** that come to mind using the technique called "brainstorming." We must not censor or criticize the ideas that arise. Any proposal should be taken advantage of, either in its entirety or varied to generate new solutions. Anything goes, even if in the beginning the possible solution seems to be completely ridiculous. It is of interest to produce many alternative solutions – the more the better.

(4) Next we implement a procedure to enable us to choose the most useful response from among all those we have produced. We must **choose the solution that provides more advantages and fewer inconveniences and risks**. We will evaluate several aspects of each one, such as the probability that this alternative solves the conflict, if we believe it will reduce anxiety or not, if it provides wellbeing, as well as the time and effort required and its long-term effects, among others. It may be helpful to assign a score to each of the solutions, using a point scale from 0 to 10.

(5) Finally, we put the solution chosen into practice and verify that it works.

Although this is a simple method, in the beginning it may seem a little artificial. However, if practiced regularly, it will soon become normal and effective. If we habitually apply this method with pencil and paper when making decisions, and assimilate it into our daily routine, it will undoubtedly assist us in our everyday functioning. It is important to try a particular solution for a reasonable time before abandoning it for another, in order to check whether it works. In the next session we will work on some real-life cases proposed by the group. We must recognize the importance not only of the execution or implementation of the chosen solution but also of the verification or confirmation of the result and how well it works. If a solution does not work, we must reassess the options or choices made.

Key points

■ Problem solving helps to reduce or eliminate negative thoughts that a person has when believing that he or she is unable to manage a situation.

■ Avoid solving any problem impulsively.

■ Before solving any problem it is necessary to analyze it and clarify its relevant processes and aspects, and thereafter to assess a number of possible solutions.

Session 16. Executive functions: solving problems

Objective

The fundamental objective of this session is to begin to put into practice the problem-solving method explained in depth in the previous session. This practice is based on real, not excessively difficult, problems which the patients may come across, with the aim of becoming familiar with the method and learning to establish the most suitable procedures to solve the problems that may arise in their daily lives.

Session procedure/guidelines for the therapist

As in all sessions, collect the task from the week before and discuss it briefly.

As a warm-up task, two rounds of verbal fluency (one in each direction) are done. For example, in the first round they might have to name different types of sports and in the second the names of professions or trades.

Before putting the problem-solving method into practice, based on real problems that the members of the group have encountered, we briefly go over the main steps to apply this method:

(1)   Problem orientation.

(2)   Problem definition and formulation.

(3)   Generation of alternatives.

(4)   Decision making.

(5)   Implementing the chosen alternatives and verification.

Thereafter, two or three volunteers are chosen to explain the problem they have prepared, and we follow the steps of the problem-solving method. Try to choose problems that may be common among the members of the group, and that are not too complex. We work on each of the problems together as a group, operatively defining the situation, proposing alternative solutions, assessing each based on the advantages, inconveniences, and risks detected, and choosing the best option. This enables the person who explained the problem to see that there are other possible ways of solving it, which may not have previously been considered, and to verify the utility and greater efficacy that the application of this method provides. A board is necessary on which each of the steps can be described, thereby making it easy for the group to follow the procedure.

Although, to begin with, this method may seem somewhat artificial, with training and practice it can become an integral part of the patients' daily routine, facilitating decision making.

To finish the session we explain the homework. It is important to review the tasks the patients bring from home, applying positive reinforcement, especially if they are making an effort to do tasks on their own (for example, if they continue with the sudokus, organizing photographs, using personal diaries or notebooks, etc.).

Homework

■   Identify stressful situations and how to manage them.

■   Continue working on news articles on the topic chosen for follow-up. If this is not possible, choose another article of interest. In the next session the material worked on, as well as the summary of the news article, should be handed in.

■   Read chapters 19, 20, and 21 of *The Little Prince* and answer the questions (see *Questions and answers on The Little Prince*, in the online material for the therapist).

Material for the patient

We will briefly go over the steps to follow in applying the problem-solving technique that we discussed in the previous session. The general objective of this technique is to help solve problems, making the most appropriate decisions. More specifically, this method intends for the person to recognize the problem at the time it starts, inhibiting any tendency to solve the problem in an impulsive way, and facilitating a wide range of possible solutions, as well as establishing the most adequate procedure to solve the problem. The result will translate into greater efficacy in coping with problems, as well as reducing stress.

The following is a summary of the steps to be taken:

(1) **Problem orientation**.

(2) **Definition and formulation of the problem**. For example, in the case of a conflict with another person, who is involved? What exactly has happened? Why does this worry us?

(3) **Generate alternatives**. To attempt to provide the maximum number of solutions possible for a situation, we must eliminate any judgment related to the quality or efficacy of any alternative. All alternatives are valid. We will try to make the alternatives as varied as possible.

(4) **Evaluation and decision making**. We will evaluate the advantages, disadvantages, and risks of each of the options suggested, so that we can make the decision we believe to be the most useful.

(5) **Implementing** the chosen alternative and **verifying** that it works.

We will use this session to provide solutions to real, simple problems described by members of the group.

Key points

When trying to solve a problem, ask yourself:

■ What am I aiming for? What are my options? Based on their pros and cons, which is the best option? What should I do first? Is it working?

Module 5. Improving communication, autonomy, and stress management

The final module integrates aspects of stress management with guidelines for diaphragmatic breathing and muscle relaxation techniques, followed by two sessions related to training in communication skills, providing some guidelines to improve conversations and enhance assertiveness and reflective listening. The penultimate session aims to reinforce social networking, supplying information concerning activities that may be done in the community.

Session 17. Managing stressful situations

Objective

We know that stress is a natural, automatic response of our organism towards situations that may be threatening. Moreover, being surrounded by an environment that constantly changes, some stress is necessary and positive in our lives for us to adapt to the continuous changes and manage the demands of the environment. Nonetheless, we also know that exposure to continued stress may lead to negative consequences, both physical and psychological, and in the case of bipolar disorder stress plays an important role as a possible trigger of relapse. In this session we therefore aim to provide the patients with information related to several psychological tools that will allow them to better manage stress and anxiety, such as promoting a change in habits and learning emotional, cognitive, and behavioral attitudes different from those that are compatible with stress.

During this session muscle relaxation is practiced, so that the patients become familiar with this technique and can continue practicing it at home.

Session procedure/guidelines for the therapist

As usual we begin the session by collecting the tasks done at home and discussing them briefly.

We then do a warm-up task. In the first round the patients should say words starting with M and in the second round words beginning with the letter R.

We start by discussing the theory, explaining what stress consists of, the main phases in which a response to stress is developed (alarm stage, resistance or adaptation stage, and exhaustion stage), and all the clinical manifestations (physical: muscle tension; and vegetative: cognitive and emotional) that may manifest when we are exposed to prolonged conditions of stress.

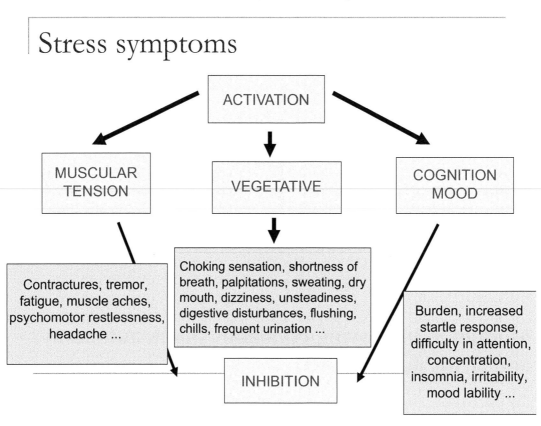

Session 17 slide 3

We propose a series of guidelines to help in coping with stress, as well as explaining different techniques, such as controlled breathing (diaphragmatic), distraction techniques, and Jacobson's progressive muscle relaxation.

Guidelines

- Modify internal aspects; do not just reduce external stressors.

- Value your achievements; do not focus on the failures.

- Rationalize the problems.

- Learn behaviors to adequately cope with stressful situations.

Session 17 slide 4

We practice diaphragmatic breathing during the session, in order for them to observe how it is done and so that they can then practice it on their own.

With regard to the distraction techniques, we emphasize that they may be useful at times of hypothymia, although they will not generally be so in states of hypomania or mania.

If further time is available, training in muscle relaxation can be performed during the session in order for them to become familar with this tool. We stress that it is important to practice relaxation daily at home until it becomes a habit.

Lastly, we explain the homework and ask a volunteer to read aloud the key point of this session.

Homework

- Practice the diaphragmatic breathing technique.
- Practice the muscle relaxation technique.
- Continue working on the news story chosen for follow-up. If this is not possible, choose another news article of interest. In the following session, the material worked on, as well as the summary of the news article, will be handed in.
- Read chapters 22, 23 and 24 of *The Little Prince* and answer the questions (see *Questions and answers on The Little Prince*, in the online material for the therapist).

Material for the patient

Stress is the natural, automatic response of our organism to threatening external situations or stimuli. These external stimuli are known as stressors, and they may be both negative and positive. Our life and surroundings are in constant change and demand continuous adaptation, and

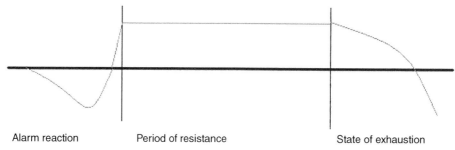

Alarm reaction   Period of resistance   State of exhaustion

Figure 4.1 The three phases of the stress response.

therefore a certain quantity of stress is necessary and positive, since this allows us to confront the demands of our environment. However, as we will see below, when it goes beyond a certain level, stress has a disorganizing effect on behavior, because the organism cannot be in a state of hyperactivity for too long.

The response to stress evolves in three phases (Figure 4.1):

■ The first phase is known as an *alarm reaction*. The physical signs and symptoms of the state of alarm are generally those of stimulation of the sympathetic nervous system. These signs include arterial hypertension, an increase in cardiac and respiratory rates, a reduction in gastrointestinal motility, pupil dilation, and increased transpiration. The person may feel nausea and loss of appetite.

■ The second phase is called the *period of resistance*. Although in this phase there are fewer physical signs than in the previous phase, the individual consumes energy in the attempt to adapt. The extent of resistance to the stressor varies from person to person, depending on the resources for confrontation of each, the total number and intensity of the stressors involved, and the external resources available such as, for example, family support, etc. This phase is characterized by a state of alertness and permanent tension.

■ The third phase takes place when the organism no longer has any capacity to adapt and enters into the *exhaustion phase*, characterized by fatigue.

Stress leads to physiological changes that are important for adaptive survival of the individual. However, if the stress is excessive and continued this may produce physical and psychiatric problems such as hypertension, asthma, insomnia, gastric problems, anxiety, depression, fatigue, and shaking. Scientific data also suggest that intense chronic stress may produce structural changes, for example in the hippocampus. As we have seen in a previous session, the hippocampus plays an important role in long-term memory. Stress may be a precursor to a depressive or manic relapse. It is therefore important to stop or relieve stress before a relapse occurs. Several techniques may help us do this.

What should we do in stress situations?

It is often difficult for a stressed person to relax, and relaxation training may sometimes have the opposite of the desired result: more irritability and tension. As shown in Figure 4.2, a vicious circle may be produced, maintaining the problem. Stress is a habit – and therefore to improve the situation, a change in habit is needed, a learning of emotional, cognitive, and behavioral conduct different from that maintaining the vicious circle.

Some important aspects are:

■ It is preferable to modify internal aspects – to try to remain "calm in the middle of the storm" – before attempting to reduce the external stressors.

■ We are frequently prone to maximizing the negative consequences of our actions and minimizing those that are positive. It may be useful to make a list of everything that is going well and which we are pleased with, so as to realistically reinforce ourselves, that is, to look at our achievements and not only at the failures.

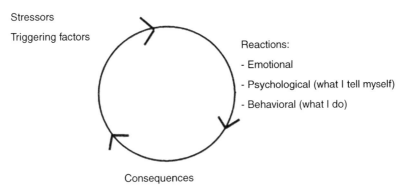

Figure 4.2 Our response to stress may result in a vicious circle in which stress is increased.

■ Rationalization of the problems. Most often we tend to overestimate the things that worry us. Relatively banal circumstances may worry us excessively compared to the really important things in life, if we do not consider them within a certain perspective.

■ Learning a behavior incompatible with stress is important. For example, if we learn to relax, we cannot be tense at the same time. To achieve this, two techniques may be useful: **diaphragmatic breathing** and **progressive muscle relaxation**.

(1) **Diaphragmatic breathing**. This can be undertaken in a number of different ways, but they all have the following in common: slowly breathe in only a little air and take this to the lower part of the lungs, displacing the diaphragm downwards. Steps:
  (a) Put one hand on your chest and the other on your stomach to ensure that you take the air to the lower part of the lungs without moving your chest.
  (b) On breathing in the air, slowly take it downwards, filling the stomach and abdomen a little without moving your chest.
  (c) Retain the air a moment in this position, counting from one to three.
  (d) Let out the air, slowly, bringing in the stomach and abdomen without moving your chest while counting from one to five.
  (e) Try to remain relaxed and let out a little more air.

(2) **Progressive muscle relaxation**. Muscle tension is one of the components of anxiety. It is an automatic involuntary mechanism, but we can learn to voluntarily control it, as occurs with breathing.

Tension and relaxation are states of the organism corresponding to two different parts of the autonomous nervous system: the **sympathetic** and the **parasympathetic**.

When we are nervous, angry, etc., we are under the control of the sympathetic nervous system, which activates the alarm system and results in physiological changes such as muscle tension.

On the other hand, when we are in a state of relaxation, it is the parasympathetic system that controls the organism, reducing cardiac and respiratory rates and diminishing muscle tension, and we feel a sensation of muscle relaxation.

Activation of the sympathetic nervous system is incompatible with that of the parasympathetic; if we are relaxed we cannot also be tense.

■ In the first phase of the exercise we will perform exercises for relaxing different muscles. We will tense up each of the groups of muscles (hands, forearms, arms, shoulders, neck, forehead, eyes, mouth, jaw, tongue, chest, abdomen, buttocks, thighs, calves, and feet) for six seconds. Then we will relax these muscles for 15 seconds. While we do the tensioning and relaxing exercises we will focus our attention on the different sensations generated in each of the states.

■ In the second phase we can mentally review each muscle group and relax any tension we feel without the need for tensing them beforehand.

On practicing these exercises, it is best to do so while wearing comfortable clothing, in a quiet place with a comfortable temperature and body position – such as lying down or seated in an armchair. Once we have learned to relax easily lying down or seated, it is convenient to get used to doing it not only seated but also in different places and situations. In this second phase, muscle relaxation can be combined with diaphragmatic breathing.

It is important to do the relaxation exercises on detecting the first signs of anxiety, before it becomes too intense.

Key points

■ Stress depends not only on external conditions but also on our personal attitudes, which are key to coping with stress and not worsening the problem.

■ It is very important to alleviate and treat stress to avoid relapses.

■ Relaxation techniques are a group of exercises that allow us to detect when our muscles are in tension and be able to relax them.

■ It is very important to practice these techniques daily at home until they become a habit.

Session 18. Training in communication skills

Objective

Communication puts human beings in contact with their environment. It is the way we make others see our wishes and our moods, as well as a way of expressing the consequences that external actions have on us. The main way we have of communicating is through spoken language, without forgetting the great importance of non-verbal communication. The act of communication is not always efficient, since not everyone develops the necessary skills. The objective of this session is to provide some guidelines for establishing appropriate communication with our environment.

Session procedure/guidelines for the therapist

Collect the task the patients had from the previous session.

Before beginning the session, we do two rounds (one in each direction) to work on verbal fluency. In the first round we might start with the word CALENDAR, and the patients have to string words together so that each word begins with the last syllable of the previous word – so in this case the next word will have to start with DAR as in DARLING, and the following word with LING as in LINGER, and so on. The second round should follow the same pattern.

We then start the session with a simple theory regarding factors that facilitate communication, as well as factors that may constitute barriers to communication between two people. We demonstrate different emotions and how they are reflected in facial expressions.

As a task to be done during the session, we show 18 photographs expressing six possible emotions (happiness, sadness, surprise, fear, anger, neutral). The photos should be observed in pairs for 15–20 seconds each, and the participants must decide which emotion is expressed in each face. Afterwards, we discuss all the results together; in the case of disagreement, we explain the clues that help to decide on one emotion or another.

Another of the activities consists of a general round in which each patient has to show some of the emotions from the previous exercise (happiness, sadness, surprise, fear, anger, or neutral) by facial expression, using the role-playing technique. The person beside them must guess what emotion they are expressing.

We continue with an explanation regarding the importance of reflective listening in communication. Thus, how we speak is not always synonymous with communication. We have to be prepared to listen, it is not an automatic process. We should do conscious, reflective listening. We list the guidelines to facilitate reflective listening and describe the attitudes which limit or obstruct it.

Reflective listening

- Show **empathy**. Try to put yourself in the place of the other.

- **Paraphrase**. This helps you to understand what the other person is saying and to check that you really understand and do not misunderstand what is being said.
  e.g., *"I see, what happened was that…", "Do you mean that you feel…?"*

- Issue **reinforcing** words or compliments.

- **Summarize**. We inform the other person of our degree of understanding or the need for further clarification.
  e.g., *"If I have not misunderstood…" " In other words, what you're saying is…", "Let's see, if I understand you…"*

Session 18 slide 29

Reflective listening

- Listening is NOT an automatic process. We must prepare for it.
- Avoid distractions.
- Do not interrupt the speaker.
- Do not judge.
- Do not offer help or premature solutions.
- Do not reject what the other person is feeling (e.g., "don't worry, it's nothing").
- Do not tell "your story" when the other person needs to talk.
- Do not counter-argue (e.g., when the other person says "I feel bad" and you respond "So do I").
- Avoid the "expert syndrome", in which you already have the answers to someone else's problem even before he or she has told you half of the story.

Session 18 slide 30

Once the theory has been completed, we ask the patients to practice reflective listening through role playing, using a dialogue. The therapists monitor the exercise and intervene if necessary, providing verbal instructions, using positive reinforcement, and reminding participants of the guidelines as necessary. The time required for this exercise is 10–15 minutes.

Approaching the end of the session, we propose a general round in which each patient acts out a profession through mimicry, while the other patients guess what it is. In a second, optional round, each patient acts out a film through mimicry.

Homework

■ Encourage the practice of reflective listening in everyday conversations with relatives, friends, neighbors, or work colleagues. Write down the advantages of the use of the new strategies and the main difficulties encountered.

■ Read the last three chapters of *The Little Prince* (see *Questions and answers on The Little Prince*, in the online material for the therapist), and work on the news article.

Material for the patient

Communication is a process that takes place between two or more people in which the participants express messages through verbal and/or non-verbal signs. Appropriate communication among people in our environment allows effective problem solving to be carried out, and leads to a reduction in stress as well as in the risk of relapses. We will discuss some of the important issues related to communication.

Non-verbal communication

Non-verbal communication is that which is carried out through our gestures, movements, looks, etc., that is, any communication that does not involve the use of words. Usually non-verbal communication is involuntary, and our emotional state has an important influence on the message conveyed. Non-verbal communication is more important than verbal communication, since, according to the experts, about 80% of what we communicate is conveyed non-verbally.

The principal components of non-verbal language, which are potentially controllable, are as follows: the look, facial expression, body position, physical contact, and the non-verbal components of speech (how things are said, including volume, tone, pitch, clarity, speed, emphasis, fluency, and pauses).

Emotion	Facial expression
Happiness	Smiling, laughing loudly, cheeks elevated, eyes squeezed between cheeks and forehead, corners of mouth raised with lips separated
Sadness	Lack of expression, descent of the corners of the mouth, downward look; if very intense, tears, shaking, and tendency to hide the face
Anger	Looking towards what has caused the anger, tension, teeth clenched, sometimes paleness or redness of the face
Fear	Eyes wide open, mouth open, generalized shaking, paleness, or sweating
Surprise	Eyes more open than usual, eyebrows elevated, lips slightly parted in the shape of an "O"

In this session we will do a group exercise to detect our ability to guess the emotional states of people by looking only at the expressions on their faces.

Verbal communication

Humans are social beings, and therefore communicating with others is necessary for us to feel well and to satisfy many other needs. However, communication sometimes presents some problems.

Misinterpretation of the message often occurs, so that the message received by the recipient is very different from what the sender intended. Our representation of reality may be different from that of other persons, and this may influence our communication.

The problem sometimes lies in that we do not transmit the message adequately and precisely, because it is not clear to us what we want to say, or because the non-verbal communication does not work in tandem with the verbal (Figure 4.3).

On occasions, we do not pay enough attention to the message we are being given. Therefore, it is very important to put **reflective listening** into practice, letting another person express the message they wish to transmit without interrupting them, paying attention, showing interest (for example, nodding with our head), and asking questions to clarify any doubts. These aspects will help us to better retain the information, and will maintain our attention.

Some **distortions** are due to environmental factors such as noises around us or even our emotional state. The mood state influences communication with those around us. The presence of depressive symptoms such as feelings of uselessness or excessive self-criticism, lack of criticism, or the suspicion that may be aroused during manic episodes, may produce a distortion in the **interpretation of the messages** received.

When the emotional levels a person manifests interfere with the interaction, it is better to interrupt the discussion and postpone it until the emotional intensity diminishes. For example, irritability affects the way messages are transmitted. For example, in the presence of the symptoms of an episode, it is better to postpone any discussion or important decision.

If you wish to express a complaint or to disagree with something, ensure that what you say is **specific** and not global, since this will facilitate solution finding. Tell the person exactly what you would like to change, or do it **in the first person** (using phrases such as "I would like ..." or "I want to ..."), looking at the person and speaking with firmness, explaining exactly what has bothered you, how it made you feel, and how to prevent this happening again in the future.

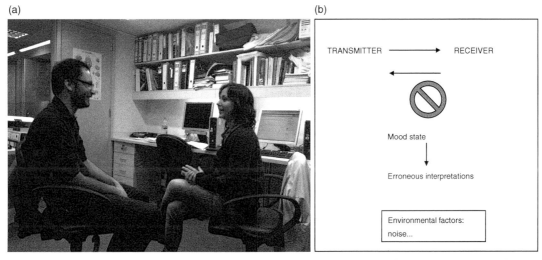

Figure 4.3 (a) Reflective listening. (b) Distortions in communication: the message received may be very different from what the transmitter intended.

In the case of possible conflictual situations, avoid "**mind reading**" and falling into erroneous interpretations of the message as far as possible. It is always better to directly ask the other person.

In some cases it may be useful to **write down** what we wish to say.

Key points

■ When we send a message, it is important to express it clearly and concisely in order for those receiving the message to understand it.

■ It is important to choose the appropriate time for the communication.

■ The role played by non-verbal communication and our mood state must be taken into account in the transmission of our messages.

Session 19. Improving communication
Objective

In this session we continue to work on different aspects of communication. We focus specifically on conversation, which constitutes the basic vehicle of communication with others. Patients often talk about difficuties in starting a conversation with another person, or in finding subjects for conversation when in a social setting. In this session we also provide basic guidelines on the style of communication called assertiveness, with which a person manifests their convictions and defends their rights without the intention of harming or affecting another. Assertiveness is a very wide concept, but in this case, because time is limited and it is covered only in this session, we restrict ourselves to some specific points such as making and refusing requests. Indeed, these are important elements in human communication, and an inability to manage these aspects well may lead to excessive anxiety and discomfort.

Session procedure/guidelines for the therapist

Discuss with the patients whether they have had any difficulty in practicing reflective listening, and if they have detected errors that they and those within their circle make in this respect.

We start, as usual, with two warm-up rounds. In the first round, for example, the patients might say words related to holidays, and in the second round they might name musical instruments.

We begin the session by practicing how to begin, maintain, and finish a conversation.

Conversation guidelines: initiating and maintaining a conversation

- Greet the other person, and introduce yourself.
- Talk about commonplace subjects to "break the ice" (e.g., weather).
- Comment on the situation in which the conversation is taking place (e.g., talking about the landscape).
- Ask if you can join the activity that the other person is doing or invite the person to join you ("Would you like to sit with us?")
- Offer praise.
- Offer something (e.g., a soft drink).
- Ask for information, help, advice, or an opinion.
- Share experiences, feelings, or other personal opinions.
- Non-verbal communication.

Session 19 slide 2

Conversation guidelines: finishing a conversation

If you are the transmitter:

- Be aware of the non-verbal language of the other person (glances at the clock, or at faces)

- Ask questions when in doubt (e.g., *"Are you in a hurry? Would you rather speak later?"*)

Session 19 slide 3

Conversation guidelines: finishing a conversation

If you are the receiver:

- Politely state that you have to go (*"Sorry, but I have to go"*).
- Summarize the conversation and express your desire to end it (*"Well, we've arranged to...."*, *"Call when there is news."*).
- Reinforce the other (*"I'm having a great time with you but I have work to do"*).
- Use non-verbal language (look at your watch or stand up).
- If you are asked if you are in a hurry, say yes, and sometimes list what you have to do.
- Postpone the conversation (*"I'm sorry but I have to go. Let's continue talking tomorrow?"*).

Session 19 slide 4

We move on to providing some guidelines on how to make and refuse requests.

Making requests

- Analyze the situation: your goals, the characteristics of the situation and of the person to whom you are going to make the request.
- The request should be reasonable, respecting the feelings and rights of the other person.
- Choose the right time to do it.
- Remember that one person is entitled to make requests and the other to reject them.
- Be careful about non-verbal language.
- Be careful of the way you make the request, and its content: be polite and realistic, formulate the request clearly, explain your interest in making this request.
- Formulate a concrete request, direct and non-contradictory.
- Do not feel obliged to explain or apologize unnecessarily.

Session 19 slide 5

Refusing requests

- Before replying, analyze the situation.

- To say NO is a right, not an obligation.

- Express refusal in a clear, brief, and polite way, without too much explanation (e.g., *"I have things to do," "I would feel bad if I did what you are requesting," "I would like to say yes but it is very inconvenient for me"*)

- Do not feel bad about yourself for giving in against your wishes.

- Do not involve yourself in situations in which you feel bad.

- **Sandwich technique.** Express something positive immediately before and after issuing the "negative" to "soften" the situation (e.g., *"Thank you for inviting me. Today does not suit me, but we could do it another day"*).

- **Scratched record technique.** Repeating an argument, over and over again, calmly.

Session 19 slide 6

Next we put the theory into practice by role playing with a spontaneous conversation (e.g., running into a neighbor at the cinema or on the metro). Depending on the time available, we can do this with one or two volunteer pairs. On finishing the exercise, we should provide positive feedback about the practice, making suggestions as to changes in behavior to produce specific modifications.

Afterwards, pairs of patients who did not do the previous role playing should practice making requests and refusing them, exchanging roles (e.g., "Ask someone to lend you a small quantity of money" or "Ask your boss to let you leave work one hour early"). At the end of the session, patients may be interested to receive more information about assertiveness. In this case, some books can be recommended (e.g., *When I Say No, I Feel Guilty* by Manuel J. Smith, 1975). This may also contribute to reinforcing the reading habit.

We end the session by reading the key points out loud.

Homework

- Write about a situation that occurred during the week in which you were able to practice the conversation guidelines. Do this so that you can explain it during the next session.

- In preparation for the next session, think about how you could realistically increase your social activities and hobbies.

- Answer some general questions on the book (see *Questions and answers on The Little Prince*, in the online material for the therapist), and make a summary of the news article.

Material for the patient

Most social interaction is based on conversation, which is an exchange of verbal and non-verbal messages between two or more people, constituting the main form of communication with others. It allows thoughts, opinions, and feelings to be shared.

The ability to initiate and maintain conversations facilitates communication and the maintenance of interpersonal relationships.

Isolation and lack of communication may predispose towards experiencing negative emotions. In contrast, communication and feelings supported by other people improves our mood state and our capacity to manage stress.

Beginning and ending a conversation

Before beginning a conversation it is useful to observe the non-verbal language of the other person, to deduce whether that person is more or less willing to converse. The best way to start a conversation depends on the situation and the context. Some examples of how to initiate a conversation are:

- Greet the other person, introduce yourself.

- Talk about clichés to break the ice ("Isn't the weather awful today?").

- Make a comment about the situation in which the conversation is taking place (for example, talk about the countryside).

- Ask if you can join an activity carried out by the other person, or if he or she would like to join yours ("Would you like to sit with us?").

- Praise some aspect of the other person's behavior or appearance, or of the situation.

- Offer the other person something (for example, a drink).

- Ask for information, help, advice, or an opinion.

- Share personal experiences, feelings, or sentiments.

- Show interest in the other person by asking a question.

Conversations have a time limit. Being skillful in social interactions includes knowing how to close them when we wish, and doing so nicely and in a friendly way. Likewise, we should be aware of the non-verbal language of the person we are conversing with, in case we observe signs of discomfort if the conversation goes on too long. Some examples to help us bring a conversation to an end are:

- State in a friendly way that you wish to finish ("Excuse me, but I have to go").

- Summarize the conversation and let the person know you wish to finish ("Well, we have agreed that . . .," "So, we'll be in touch when there is some news").

- Reinforce the other person ("I'm having a great time with you, but I have some work I have to do").

- Use non-verbal language (for example, look at your watch or stand up).

- If you are asked if you are in a hurry, say yes, and sometimes explain what you have to do.

- Adjourn the conversation ("Sorry but I have to go – maybe we could continue talking tomorrow?").

Making and refusing requests

Making requests of others is a natural thing to do, since we are social beings and a large proportion of our goals are related to the behavior of other people. The fear of rejection often blocks us and impedes making a request adequately, thereby not allowing us to fulfill our objectives.

Making requests involves asking favors, asking for help, and asking another person to change their behavior. We have the right to ask for what we want provided the rights of others are not violated, although we also have to keep in mind that the other person has the right to refuse based on their wishes and preferences.

Firstly, before making a request, it is useful to analyze our objectives as well as the characteristics of the situation and the person to whom we are going to make the request. We should take into account the following guidelines:

- Formulate a reasonable request, which respects the feelings and rights of the other person.

- Choose the opportune time to make the request.

- Remember that one person has the right to make a request, and the other person has the right to refuse.

- Be careful with non-verbal language.

- Be careful with the content of the request and the way it is expressed. Be polite, be realistic, make it clear, explain your interest in the request, etc.

- Formulate the request in a concrete, direct, and non-confrontational way.

- Do not feel obliged to give explanations or ask for unnecessary apologies.

You should also be able to refuse requests made of you by others in a natural way without feeling guilty for having done so. It is important not to get involved in situations that would make us feel bad or angry with the other person or with ourselves. On refusing a request, the following questions should be taken into account:

- Before answering, analyze the situation; make sure you have understood adequately.

- Saying **"no"** is a right, not an obligation.

- Express the refusal clearly, briefly, and in a polite way, but not beating around the bush or giving too many explanations ("I have things I have to do," "I would feel bad if I did what you ask of me," "I would like to say yes, but I really can't...").

- Do not become involved in situations in which you would feel bad.

- **Sandwich technique**. Express something positive immediately before and after sending the "negative" message, to soften the situation, which may be upsetting ("Thanks for inviting me. Today I can't, but we could arrange to meet another day").

- **Scratched record technique**. Repeat an argument over and over again without losing your calm.

- Do not get upset with yourself for having given in against your wishes.

In this session, we will work on initiating conversations and how to accept and refuse requests through the role-playing technique. Role playing is a technique in which a situation from real life is simulated. In this case, we will do role playing about a conversation with a member of the family or a friend. On practicing this technique we should adopt the role of a specific person and create a situation as if it were real.

The objective is to imagine the way to act and the decisions we would make in each of the different situations. We can exchange the roles, and this will help us put ourselves into the place of the other person, practice, think about how we would act, what we would say, etc. This technique will allow us to work on empathy (putting ourselves in the place of another) and comprehension. It will also allow us to solve conflicts and assume responsibility for decision making.

Key points

- Improving communication can lead to a reduction in stress, and can prevent relapses.

- Improving our communication skills helps us with our social functioning and interpersonal relationships.

Session 20. Improving autonomy and functioning

Objective

The objective of this second-last session is to facilitate and empower patient autonomy to a maximum. In particular, we attempt to reinforce the social network, providing them with information concerning activities that may be done in their neighborhood, and also working on their autonomy in activities that are perhaps done by the relatives but which they could do by themselves.

Session procedure/guidelines for the therapist

In the first warm-up round, the patients say words related to sports, and in the second round, words starting with the syllable *re*.

In this session, we invite the social worker of the center to provide detailed information about the volunteer services, civic centers, and libraries, as well as about the occupational situation (pensions, disability, etc.)

In the case of a center without a social worker, collect as much information as possible for the patients, in order to facilitate an increase in their social, occupational, and voluntary activities and hobbies.

Another aspect covered is to learn to better manage money through the control of expenses and making balanced purchases. In general, we will empower autonomy, involving the patients in doing the maximum number of tasks possible by themselves: control of medication, mobile phone applications, using a computer, how to consult email, doing administrative work, etc.

At the end of the session we remind the members of the group to bring back the book they have read and the summaries they have prepared, because we will be devoting some time to this in the last session.

We read the key points and hand out the information concerning addresses and telephone numbers that the social worker (or ourselves) has prepared.

At the end of the session, depending on the time available, an extra 10–15 minutes of individual attention will be given to each patient.

Homework

- Once the book has been finished, write a personal opinion about it, which will be collected in the last session. If any patient is a little behind in this respect he/she can have this session to finish the book.

Material for the patient

Psychosocial functioning includes several aspects, such as the capacity to work, live independently, study, enjoy leisure time, and have a stable social network.

Sometimes, as a consequence of the course of the disease, patients are unable to continue working in their usual role and must ask for temporary leave or in some cases opt for a disability pension. At this time, apart from the clinical aspects related to the disease itself, aspects of psychosocial functioning come into play. The social circle of the patient may be reduced if they do not work, and a distancing from friends occurs. People in the patient's social circle often view some of the symptoms of the disease with uncertainty, not knowing how to act.

Because of the relapses, some people with bipolar disorder may experience a significant reduction in activity in general. If the time of recovery between episodes is somewhat prolonged, many of the routines of daily life may be altered. This may lead to a vicious circle in which the patient becomes "shut up" at home with a very sedentary routine, with negative consequences for his or her physical health, on top of the damage to emotional health that arises from the drastic reduction in external stimuli. This situation favors the appearance of thoughts and emotions of a more depressive nature, as well as reduced motivation for interacting with the external world.

On the other hand, a patient's family is a very important source of support, but they may often adopt an attitude of excessive watchfulness and overprotection, interpreting all the reactions of the patient as if they were the product of the disease, and not allowing the patient to develop autonomy. It is important to reach an intermediate point at which the disorder is accepted and expectations of social and occupational functioning are restructured, while at the same time encouraging patients to do things by themselves to potentiate their independence (being responsible for the shopping, arranging an appointment with the doctor, organizing their own medication, managing their own money with good control of expenses, learning to use new technology such as the internet or a mobile phone, etc.). In evaluating which activities or tasks should be carried out, it is important to strike a balance between overloading the patient and leaving him or her inactive, with very little to do.

It is of great importance to construct a solid social environment – a stable social network. Sometimes a patient association can help with this function, as can day centers, or taking courses on topics that interest us at a neighborhood civic center to stimulate intellectual aspects, or participating in volunteer groups or activities, doing jobs according to our abilities, etc. In this way, better social integration and greater wellbeing may be achieved.

Key points

■ The acquisition of social skills increases self-confidence, while also considerably reducing levels of stress.

Session 21. Final session: review of useful strategies

Objective

This is the last session. These six months of weekly contact have been very important for the patients, making the closure of this circle in which they have participated and worked all this time very relevant. They should not have the sensation that all is finished, but rather that they can remain in contact with us if they need to. We should give them our contact information. We should thank them for participating in the group and give them a certificate of participation in the Functional Remediation Course.

Session procedure/guidelines for the therapist

In the first of two warm-up rounds, the patients say words related to professions, and in the second round, words starting with the letter M.

We then answer any questions on the content of the previous sessions, asking them their opinion about the book and the questions they had to answer on its content.

We ask their opinion as to whether they believe that their participation in the course has made any improvement in some aspects of cognition and functioning. Likewise, we ask them their opinion as to what aspects of the intervention could be improved.

We thank the group and say goodbye.

We provide the patients our addresses in order to easily locate us in the hospital.

They are given a sheet on which to evaluate the course.

Group evaluation

	Yes	No
■ Did the program meet your expectations?	☐	☐

If not, which aspects would you improve?

_____

_____

	Yes	No
■ Did you feel comfortable?	☐	☐

■ Overall evaluation of the program

☹ _____ ☺

0   1   2   3   4   5   6   7   8   9   10

Session 21 slide 4

Material for the patient

Today is the last day of this course. If you are reading the content of this last session this means that you have completed the program.

You have participated in an innovative project, since this is the first functional rehabilitation program designed specifically for people with bipolar disorder. We have tailored the sessions to meet your specific needs, in the environment in which you find yourselves, taking into account our experience in the treatment of bipolar disorder.

The overall objective of these sessions was, on the one hand, to improve aspects of cognitive function such as attention, concentration, memory, and the executive functions (including problem-solving techniques and the management of stress) and, on the other hand, to improve the psychosocial functioning of each one of you. Better management of cognitive problems, making use of the different guidelines and strategies presented in the course of the sessions, will surely help to improve your autonomy and quality of life.

We hope we have fulfilled your expectations, and that we have been able to equip you with some useful tools and show you how to continue applying them in your everyday life once these sessions are finished. Our general evaluation of the sessions, together with your observations and suggestions, will allow us in the future to "polish up" those aspects of the program that require it.

We wish to thank you for your active participation, and congratulate you on having completed the program. We encourage you to continue putting into practice the techniques and strategies that we have worked on over the past few months, in order to consolidate and integrate them into your daily lives.

Appendix 1

Functioning Assessment Short Test (FAST)

Questionnaire

To what extent is the patient experiencing difficulties in each of the following areas? Ask the patient about each of the 24 areas of possible difficulty in functioning and score according to the following scale: (0) no difficulty, (1) mild difficulty, (2) moderate difficulty, (3) severe difficulty.

AUTONOMY

1. Taking responsibility for a household   (0) (1) (2) (3)
2. Living on your own   (0) (1) (2) (3)
3. Doing the shopping   (0) (1) (2) (3)
4. Taking care of yourself (physical aspects, hygiene)   (0) (1) (2) (3)

OCCUPATIONAL FUNCTIONING

5. Holding down a paid job   (0) (1) (2) (3)
6. Accomplishing tasks as quickly as necessary   (0) (1) (2) (3)
7. Working in the field in which you were educated (0) (1) (2) (3)
8. Occupational earnings   (0) (1) (2) (3)
9. Managing the expected work load   (0) (1) (2) (3)

COGNITIVE FUNCTIONING

10. Ability to concentrate on a book or film   (0) (1) (2) (3)
11. Ability to make mental calculations   (0) (1) (2) (3)
12. Ability to solve a problem adequately   (0) (1) (2) (3)
13. Ability to remember newly learned names   (0) (1) (2) (3)
14. Ability to learn new information   (0) (1) (2) (3)

FINANCIAL ISSUES

15. Managing your own money   (0) (1) (2) (3)
16. Spending money in a balanced way   (0) (1) (2) (3)

INTERPERSONAL RELATIONSHIPS

17. Maintaining a friendship or friendships   (0) (1) (2) (3)
18. Participating in social activities   (0) (1) (2) (3)
19. Having good relationships with people close to you (0) (1) (2) (3)
20. Living together with your family   (0) (1) (2) (3)
21. Having satisfactory sexual relationships   (0) (1) (2) (3)
22. Being able to defend your interests   (0) (1) (2) (3)

LEISURE TIME

23. Doing exercise or participating in sport   (0) (1) (2) (3)
24. Having hobbies or personal interests   (0) (1) (2) (3)

Description of the scale

The FAST is a simple instrument, easy to administer in a short time (3–6 minutes). It was developed for the clinical evaluation of difficulties presented by psychiatric illness, particularly bipolar disorder (Rosa et al., 2007). One of the advantages of the FAST is that it is applicable in both clinical practice and research settings. It is useful in clinical trials to evaluate the functioning of individuals receiving different treatments. The FAST is a scale designed for ongoing assessment of functioning, and it is able to evaluate minimal changes achieved by different treatments, including improvements and worsening of symptoms (depressive, manic phases).

The 24 items of the scale are divided among six specific areas of functioning: autonomy, occupational functioning, cognitive functioning, financial issues, interpersonal relationships, and leisure time.

(1) Autonomy refers to the patient's capacity for doing things alone and taking his/her own decisions.

(2) Occupational functioning refers to the capacity to maintain a paid job, efficiency of performing tasks at work, working in the field in which the patient was educated, and earning according to the level of the employment position.

(3) Cognitive functioning is related to the ability to concentrate, performing simple mental calculations, solving problems, learning and recall of new information.

(4) Financial issues involve the capacity to manage finances and spend in a balanced way.

(5) Interpersonal relationships refer to relations with friends and family, involvement in social activities, sexual relationships, and the ability to defend one's own interests.

(6) Leisure time refers to the capability to perform physical activities (sport, exercise) and the enjoyment of hobbies.

■ The scale is interviewer-administered.

■ The studied time frame refers to the last 15 days before assessment.

■ The scale provides a score for each item.

■ The clinician has to evaluate the limitations presented by the patient, taking into account the expected functioning of a person of the same sex, age, and sociocultural status.

Translations

The scale is available in six languages: Spanish, English, Portuguese, German, Italian, and French.

Instructions for the assessment

A standardized administration of the FAST for all patients is important. In this way, differences in answers due to differences in administration will be avoided. It is important to make sure that the results are standardized.

A good and clear introduction of the FAST is fundamental. Before starting with the assessment, the interviewer should explain to the patient the purpose of the evaluation and also answer his/her questions. The following points have to be included in the introduction:

■ Name and affiliation of the interviewer.

■ If he/she is a doctor or an investigator.

■ The questionnaire is important as a means of obtaining data with respect to bipolar disorder.

■ The participation of the patient is voluntary and fundamental for the continuation of the examination/diagnostic phase.

■ It is important that each question is answered as accurately and truthfully as possible.

The questions must be read out exactly as they are presented in the questionnaire (above). The question: "To what extent is the patient experiencing difficulties in the following area?" has to be asked before each question. Questions should be repeated when the patient is in doubt or when it appears that the patient did not hear the question well. Additional questions can be asked, and information obtained through a partner or close relative should be considered. As part of the interviewer-administered scale of objective evaluation, the score must reflect the clinician's evaluation and not necessarily the literal description given by the patient.

Scores

The FAST provides an overall score of the patient's functioning and a score for each of the following domains: autonomy, occupational functioning, cognitive functioning, financial issues, interpersonal relationships, and leisure time. Each individual item is scored from 0 to 3. The global score is obtained by adding up the scores of all the items. The higher the score, the more serious the difficulties.

The criteria for the scores are:

(0)   No difficulty: the functioning of the patient is in accordance with the norms of the reference group or sociocultural context; there are no difficulties at any moment.

(1)   Mild difficulty: minimal difficulties, there are deviations from the norm in one or more of the activities or functions. The patient can be considered as having slight disabilities.

(2)   Moderate difficulty: there are strong deviations from the norm in most of the activities and functions. The patient can be considered as having moderate or serious disabilities most of the time.

(3)   Severe difficulty: maximal difficulties, the deviation of the norm has reached a critical point. The patient is considered to have serious disabilities.

Details of scoring on each of the six domains

Autonomy

1. Taking responsibility for a household

Ask if the patient is able to identify and to maintain basic management of the household. The activities could be cleaning the dishes, clothes washing, cooking, changing a light bulb. Some people are not used to doing household tasks because they receive help from other people (e.g., mother or partner) to do so. Nevertheless, it is important to know if the patient is capable of fulfilling tasks in the household or arranging for somebody else to undertake the household tasks. Enquire about other activities that identify autonomy. For example, ask: "If your partner is ill, will you be able to cope with the household tasks?"

(0)   No difficulty. The functioning of the patient is in accordance with the norms of the reference group or the sociocultural context.

(1)   Mild difficulty. The patient can do the tasks with a minimum of difficulties: for example, sometimes the patient does the tasks slowly or sometimes he/she cannot finish them.

(2)   Moderate difficulty. Most of the time, the patient is not able to do the tasks because he/she cannot identify what has to be done. The patient is not able to finish the daily tasks alone and he/she depends on the assistance of other people.

(3)   Severe difficulty. The patient is completely unable to apply him/herself to the task, and requires the help of other people all the time.

2. Living on your own

Ask if the patient is capable of living on his/her own, without the help of a partner, mother, or others. If the patient lives with other people, it is important to find out if he/she could live alone (e.g., the patient has sufficient autonomy and would feel safe to live alone). For example, ask: "Do you think you are able to live alone?"

(0)   No difficulty. The patient is able to live alone. The functioning of the patient is in accordance with the norms of the reference group or the sociocultural context.

(1)   Mild difficulty. The patient is able or would be able to live alone most of the time. Possibly, sometimes the patient experiences some difficulties in organizing and needs help from other people.

(2)   Moderate difficulty. Most of the time the patient has moderate difficulty in living alone, and needs help from other people. Patients who live alone but need other people to manage their everyday lives such as doing the shopping or cleaning up the house. For example, patients who live near their family and are depending on them for managing their responsibilities.

(3)   Severe difficulty. The patient is completely unable to live alone. The patient depends on the assistance of other people all the time. Patients are not able to take medications or clean the house.

3. Doing the shopping

Ask about shopping in the supermarket or bakery. It is important to find out if the patient has the autonomy to do the shopping, to organize a list of products, to administer his/her budget without requiring help from other people.

(0)   No difficulty. The functioning of the patient is in accordance with the norms of the reference group or the sociocultural context.

(1)   Mild difficulty. The patient is able to do the shopping with minimal difficulties, e.g., sometimes the patient fails to complete the shopping or it requires significant effort to do so. Sometimes the patient is not able to take the initiative to do the shopping or to organize purchases.

(2)   Moderate difficulty. Most of the time the patient is not able to organize purchases or do the shopping, and needs help from other people. The patient is not able to take the initiative to do the shopping or to organize purchases.

(3)   Severe difficulty. The patient is incapable of doing the shopping or going to the supermarket or bakery.

4. Taking care of yourself (physical aspects, hygiene)

Ask about difficulties with taking a shower, shaving, combing the hair, dressing suitably. In this question the evaluation of the interviewer is very important.

(0)   No difficulty. Suitable physical appearance.

(1)   Mild difficulty. The physical aspects are slightly neglected (for example, the patient needs to shave, needs to dress suitably, his/her clothing is inadequate even though he/she has good hygiene).

(2)   Moderate difficulty. Most of the time the physical aspects are inadequate for the occasion (e.g., lack of shaving, problems in combing the hair, dirty clothes, unpleasant smell, bad hygiene), leading to discomfort or even rejection by close people. In this situation, the patient is able to take care of him/herself although he/she does not do so regularly.

(3)   Severe difficulty. The physical aspects are totally inadequate for the occasion, and personal hygiene is only possible with help from other people.

Occupational functioning

Inpatients, patients receiving invalidity benefit, or people requiring sick leave because of their psychiatric illness must receive scores of 3.

Students should be evaluated according to their fulfillment of their studies. Students who are still studying even though they would be expected to be working, given their age, should receive a score of 3.

Housewives should be considered as active workers when this was the situation prior to illness onset. However, when this situation is due to the psychiatric illness, the score should be 3. Housewives should be evaluated according to the fulfillment of their responsibilities.

Patients in social employment programs should be scored 3 on items 5 and 8. Items 6, 7, and 9 should be scored based on their responsibilities. For example, depressed patients who are participating in a social rehabilitation program in order to integrate into the community should receive a score of 3.

5. Holding down a paid job

Ask if the patient is employed, and what type of work he/she does. All types of paid jobs (formal/informal) must be considered here, since the patients earn money in accordance with their level of education. This item also assesses whether with the patient's salary can cover all his/her needs.

(0)   No difficulty. The patient has a paid job and is able to maintain a mean income per month. Retired patients score 0.

(1)   Mild difficulty. The patient maintains a job, but reduces his/her working day, resulting in a decreased income and some difficulties in maintaining economic responsibilities.

(2)   Moderate difficulty. The patient is not able to maintain his/her job for long periods of time, e.g., patients that change jobs or have had short sick leaves once or twice within the last 12 months. This situation results in economic consequences and creates difficulty for the patient in maintaining his/her responsibilities.

(3)   Severe difficulty. The patient is unable to undertake employment. Patients who have lost their jobs because of the illness, patients receiving invalidity benefit, patients in unpaid social employment programs, inpatients or patients who have taken sick leaves several times (more than twice) during the last 12 months, and job seekers all fall within this score category.

Note: Students and housewives/house-husbands must receive scores equal to 0.

6. Accomplishing tasks as quickly as necessary

Ask about the speed at which the employed patient is able to accomplish tasks at work. In other words, it is important to evaluate whether the speed is the same as or slower than other people in the same position. The key is to find out if the illness affects the performance at work in terms of speed. Students should be evaluated according to the fulfillment of their studies, and housewives should be evaluated according to the fulfillment of their responsibilities.

(0)   No difficulty. The functioning of the patient is according to the norms of the reference group or the sociocultural context.

(1)   Mild difficulty. In general, the patient finishes the tasks with minimal difficulty and, although sometimes perhaps slower than others, completes his/her tasks efficaciously.

(2)   Moderate difficulty. Most of the time the patient is not able to finish his/her tasks as quickly as necessary.

(3)   Severe difficulty. The patient is unemployed or is totally insufficient in terms of speed. Assign this score to patients who have lost their jobs because of illness, patients receiving invalidity benefit, patients who have taken sick leaves because of the illness, and inpatients.

Note: For retired patients, answer this question in respect of the last period of time in which they were employed.

7. Working in the field in which you were educated

Ask if the patient works in the field in which he/she was educated. It is important to find out if the patient works according to his/her level of education or if there is a gap between the level of education and the employment position that indicates a sign of disability or handicap.

(0) No difficulty. The functioning of the patient is in accordance to the norms of the reference group or the sociocultural context.

(1) Mild difficulty. The patient works in the same area of education, but not at his/her level of education (for example: if he/she is an architect but works as a graphic designer).

(2) Moderate difficulty. The patient does not work in the same area of education. For example, if he/she is an engineer but works as a waiter/waitress.

(3) Severe difficulty. The patient is unemployed or shows obvious signs of his/her disability in the workplace. Patients who have lost their jobs because of the illness, patients receiving invalidity benefit, patients in unpaid social employment programs, patients who have taken sick leaves, and inpatients should receive scores of 3.

Note: For retired patients, answer this question in respect of the last period of time in which they performed employment.

This item does not apply to students and housewives/house-husbands, who should score 0.

8. Occupational earnings

Ask if the patient is paid according to the position that he/she occupies, in comparison to his/her colleagues.

(0) No difficulty. The functioning of the patient is in accordance with the norms of the reference group or the sociocultural context.

(1) Mild difficulty. The patient earns slightly less than other people in the same position.

(2) Moderate difficulty. The patient earns less than other people in same position.

(3) Severe difficulty. Unemployed. Patients who have lost their jobs because of the illness, patients receiving invalidity benefit, patients in unpaid social employment programs, patients who have taken sick leave because of the illness, and inpatients score 3.

Note: For retired patients, answer this question in respect of the last period of time in which they were employed. Students and housewives/house-husbands score according to the clinician's evaluation, considering the score of item 8 independently of item 7.

9. Managing the expected work load

Ask about the performance of the patient in the tasks at work. Does he/she have the capacity to initiate and finish expected activities? Students and housewives/house-husbands should be evaluated according to the fulfillment of their studies/responsibilities.

(0) No difficulty. The performance of the patient is in accordance with the norms of the reference group or the sociocultural context.

(1) Mild difficulty. The patient functions with minimal difficulty. He/she is able to fulfill his/her goals and carry out the proposed activities in a sufficient way.

(2) Moderate difficulty. The patient shows a lower performance than the reference group. Most of the time, he/she is unable to fulfill a complete day of work and/or to finish daily tasks.

(3)   Severe difficulty. Unemployed. Patients who have lost their jobs because of the disease, patients receiving invalidity benefit, patients who have taken sick leave because of the illness, and inpatients all score 3.

Note: For retired patients, answer this question in respect of the last period of time in which they were employed.

Cognitive functioning

10. Ability to concentrate on a book or film

Ask if the patient is able to concentrate on reading a book or watching a film or soap opera, and if he/she is able to remember what he/she had read before or if he/she is able to comment on the movie that he/she had seen. If the patient does not read or does not watch films, try to find out if this originated from a concentration problem.

(0)   No difficulty. The concentration of the patient is in accordance with the norms of the reference group or the sociocultural context.

(1)   Mild difficulty. The patient carries out the intellectual activities with minimal difficulties. Although he/she is slightly distracted, most of the time the patient is able to concentrate, but sometimes has difficulties in understanding a film, or reading a book, etc.

(2)   Moderate difficulty. Most of the time the patient performs the intellectual activities with effort: for example, he/she needs to read an article in the newspaper several times, is not able to watch a film until the end or has difficulties in concentrating, or is not able to understand a soap opera even though he/she follows it daily.

(3)   Severe difficulty. The patient is not able to start reading or to understand the plot of a film or soap opera.

11. Ability to make mental calculations

Ask about difficulties with simple arithmetic, such as calculating the change while shopping in the supermarket. The important thing is to assess the capacity for dealing with calculations of addition and subtraction and evaluate if there is an alteration in his/her capacity to make mental calculations because of the illness.

(0)   No difficulty. The functioning of the patient is in accordance with the norms of the reference group or the sociocultural context.

(1)   Mild difficulty. Minimal difficulties performing simple mental calculations, but he/she can do it most of the time.

(2)   Moderate difficulty. The patient has a relevant decrement in his/her ability to make simple mental calculations. The patient is unable to do it most of the time.

(3)   Severe difficulty. The patient is totally unable to undertake simple mental calculations.

12. Ability to solve a problem adequately

Ask how the patient deals with daily problems and simple problems in general. For example, ask the patient if he/she is able to deal with administration procedures, such as what to do if his/her wallet is stolen or if he/she misses a train, or if he/she is able to find medical assistance when it is necessary.

(0)   No difficulty. The patient is able to solve daily problems.

(1)   Mild difficulty. In general, the patient is able to solve a problem alone but sometimes he/she needs other people's help.

(2)   Moderate difficulty. Most of the time the patient needs other people's help.

(3)   Severe difficulty. Unable to solve basic problems. The patient always needs help from other people.

13. Ability to remember newly learned names

Ask if the patient is able to remember the names of people he/she met recently (for example when he/she is introduced to somebody), telephone numbers, or the supermarket list, or if he/she needs a list to remember the products he/she has to buy in the market.

(0) No difficulty. The patient is able to remember newly learned names and new information.

(1) Mild difficulty. In general, the patient has a slight decrement in his/her ability to remember names/lists of products.

(2) Moderate difficulty. Most of the time, the patient has marked decrement in his/her ability to remember names or new information.

(3) Severe difficulty. The patient is never able to remember names/new information.

14. Ability to learn new information

Ask if the patient is able to learn things, for example, a new task at work, taking and remembering a new route, food recipes, how to operate household electric devices (DVD, MP3, Internet). If the patient is not interested in learning new information, try to find out if this is caused by having difficulties in understanding new information.

(0) No difficulty. The patient is able to learn and recall new information.

(1) Mild difficulty. In general the patient needs minimal effort in learning and recalling, due to slight difficulties in encoding new information.

(2) Moderate difficulty. The patient is able to learn simple information with maximal effort, e.g., needing several explanations.

(3) Severe difficulty. The patient is totally unable to learn new information.

Financial issues

15. Managing your own money

Ask if the patient has economic independence, and find out if he/she is able to manage his/her income during the month: for example, if he/she is able to buy according to his/her budget. Ask if the patient is able to support someone with their own money.

(0) No difficulty. The patient is able to manage his/her money adequately during the month.

(1) Mild difficulty. Most of the time the patient is able to manage expenses within the month, and only experiences minimal difficulties with some momentary inadequate management.

(2) Moderate difficulty. The patient is able to manage or organize his/her finances/earnings, but needs constant help and supervision from others.

(3) Severe difficulty. The patient cannot manage his/her income and does not have a perception of the value of money. He/she is dependent on others.

16. Spending money in a balanced way

Ask if the patient is able to make balanced purchases adjusted to his/her budget, without excessive spending.

(0) No difficulty. The patient is able to manage money in a balanced way.

(1) Mild difficulty. Most of the time the patient is able to do the shopping appropriately, but sometimes he/she can make inappropriate purchases.

(2) Moderate difficulty. The patient is able to undertake balanced purchases but needs constant supervision from others.

(3) Severe difficulty. The patient does not have an adequate perception of the value of money, spending a lot of money; he/she is totally dependent on other people.

Interpersonal relationships

17. Maintaining a friendship or friendships

Ask the patient if he/she has friends, if he/she is able to maintain these friendships, if he/she is able to make new friendships. It is important to evaluate if the interpersonal relationships are not restricted to the family environment.

(0)   No difficulty. The patient is able to maintain a friendship or friendships (at least once per week), or he/she is able to make new friendships without effort.

(1)   Mild difficulty. The patient is able to maintain a friendship (at least once every two weeks), but he/she is only able to make new friendships with some effort.

(2)   Moderate difficulty. The patient is able to maintain his/her friendships (at least once every two weeks), but he/she is only able to make new friendships with maximum effort.

(3)   Severe difficulty. The patient does not have friends, does not make friends. The patient lives predominantly isolated inside a family environment.

18. Participating in social activities

Ask the patient if he/she participates in social/group meetings or social activities: birthdays, weddings, barbecues, and meetings.

(0)   No difficulty. The patient is able to participate in a range of social activities.

(1)   Mild difficulty. The patient participates in social meetings. Possibly he/she is participating in social meetings but he/she remains in the background and the interaction takes some effort. The patient is more reserved, avoiding relationships; for example, the patient does not participate in conversations or leaves earlier than other people.

(2)   Moderate difficulty. Most of the time the patient is unable to participate in group meetings, weddings, or birthday parties. He/she has the tendency to be in the family environment.

(3)   Severe difficulty. The patient does not have any social activities apart from within the family setting. During family activities the patient has the tendency to be isolated.

19. Having good relationships with people close to you

Ask the patient about his/her relations with other people outside the family. For example, is he/she able to initiate or to maintain a conversation and have a friendly relationship with people such as neighbors and colleagues? Note: do not consider relationships with family members in this question.

(0)   No difficulty. The patient is able to have good relationships with people close to him/her.

(1)   Mild difficulty. The patient is able to maintain a conversation and has a friendly relationship with people close to him/her with minimal effort.

(2)   Moderate difficulty. The patient has moderate difficulties in maintaining a conversation and having a friendly relationship with people close to him/her. In general, the patient has conflicts with people and avoids the possibility of having interpersonal relationships.

(3)   Severe difficulty. The patient is not able to establish any relations with people around him/her.

20. Living together with your family

Ask the patient about relations with his/her family in general. If there are any problems with a family member, the score should at least be 1.

(0)   No difficulty. The patient has no difficulty in living together with his/her family.

(1)   Mild difficulty. The patient has some difficulties with one or more family members.

(2) Moderate difficulty. The patient has important conflicts with the family, leading to problems in living together with his/her family.

(3) Severe difficulty. The patient causes fights within the family setting. The patient gets isolated from his/her environment.

21. Having satisfactory sexual relationships

Ask if sexual relationships are satisfactory. It is more important to evaluate the level of satisfaction than the frequency of sexual relationships. Patients who are inactive sexually, but who are satisfied with their sexual condition, should receive a score of 0.

(0) Patient has satisfactory sexual relationships.

(1) Patient has slightly unsatisfactory sexual relationships.

(2) Patient has moderately unsatisfactory sexual relationships.

(3) Patient has totally unsatisfactory sexual relationships.

22. Being able to defend your interests

Ask if the patient is able to articulate or express his/her opinions and ideas and to defend his/her interests, as well as to say "no" when it is necessary.

(0) No difficulty. The patient is able to defend his/her interests.

(1) Mild difficulty. The patient is able to articulate or to express his/her own interests and put limitations when it is necessary. However, sometimes he/she cannot do it.

(2) Moderate difficulty. Most of the time the patient is unable to articulate or to express his/her own interests.

(3) Severe difficulty. The patient does not succeed in defending his/her ideas and opinions.

Leisure time

23. Doing exercise or participating in sport

Ask about whether or not there are problems with daily physical activities such as walking, swimming, cycling, or playing soccer. Sometimes the patient can do physical activities such as walking for 15 minutes to get to the bus stop every day. This item should also consider the physical activity done related to his/her profession (builder, painter, etc.). Situations that require momentary effort should not be considered as physical activity. This item should be evaluated according to level of regular physical activity.

(0) No difficulty. The patient does a regular physical activity in his/her routine and he/she understands the necessity for it.

(1) Mild difficulty. The patient is able to do exercise or sports with some difficulty. However, sometimes he/she does not play sport or exercise.

(2) Moderate difficulty. The patient is not able to continue a sport or performs only few physical activities. He/she is almost physically inactive.

(3) Severe difficulty. The patient is not able to perform any physical activity. The patient leads a complete sedentary lifestyle.

24. Having hobbies or personal interests

Ask about hobbies: for example, visiting friends, playing cards or other games, going to the cinema, reading, etc. Ask if the patient is able to enjoy his/her hobbies.

(0)   No difficulty. In general, the patient has hobbies and enjoys them.

(1)   Mild difficulty. The patient is able to enjoy hobbies, although he/she has some difficulties.

(2)   Moderate difficulty. Most of the time the patient is unable to enjoy his/her hobbies, or performs scarcely any activities related to them.

(3)   Severe difficulty. The patient does not have hobbies or is not able to enjoy them.

Appendix

Appendix 2

Neuropsychological battery

Neurocognitive domain	Task/subtest
Intelligence quotient (IQ)	Estimated by the **Wechsler Adult Intelligence Scale (WAIS-III) vocabulary subtest**
The Processing Speed Index	**Symbol search (WAIS-III)**
	Digit Symbol Coding (WAIS-III)
Frontal executive functions	**The computerized Wisconsin Card Sorting Test (WCST)**
	Stroop Color–Word Interference Test (SCWT). Assesses interference resistance.
	FAS and animal naming (Controlled Oral Word Association Test). Assesses verbal fluency.
Attention and working memory	**Trail Making Test (TMT)**. Assesses mainly attention and visuomotor speed.
	Continuous Performance Test (CPT-II). For the assessment of sustained attention and psychomotor speed.
Working memory	**Arithmetic (WAIS-III)**. Subject is asked to mentally resolve a number of numerical problems, with a time limit.
	Digits forward and backwards (WAIS-III)
	Letter–Number Sequencing (WAIS-III). Consists of chains of mixed letters and numbers that are presented orally to the subject, who must first repeat the numbers in ascending order and then the letters in alphabetical order.
Verbal learning and memory	**Logical Memory Scale (WMS-III)**. Evaluates the immediate and delayed recall of two short stories and the performance of a recognition task.
	California Verbal Learning Test (CVLT) to assess verbal learning and memory.
Visual memory	**Rey–Osterreith Complex Figure Test (ROCF)**. Evaluates visuoconstructive and visuospatial ability and visual memory, because after a few minutes the subject must return to reproduce the figure in the absence of the model.

2

Appendix

References

Albus, M., Hubmann, W., Ehrenberg, C., *et al.* 1996. Neuropsychological impairment in first-episode and chronic schizophrenic patients. *Eur Arch Psychiatry Clin Neurosci* **246**, 249–55.

Altshuler, L., Mintz, J., & Leight, K. 2002. The Life Functioning Questionnaire (LFQ): a brief, gender-neutral scale assessing functional outcome. *Psychiatry Res* **112**, 161–82.

Altshuler, L.L., Post, R.M., Black, D.O., *et al.* 2006. Subsyndromal depressive symptoms are associated with functional impairment in patients with bipolar disorder: results of a large, multisite study. *J Clin Psychiatry* **67**, 1551–60.

Anaya, C., Martínez-Arán, A., Ayuso-Mateos, J.L., *et al.* 2012. A systematic review of cognitive remediation for schizo-affective and affective disorders. *J Affect Disord* **142**, 13–21.

Antila, M., Tuulio-Henriksson, A., Kieseppa, T., *et al.* 2007. Cognitive functioning in patients with familial bipolar I disorder and their unaffected relatives. *Psychol Med* **37**, 679–87.

Arts, B., Jabben, N., Krabbendam, L., & van Os, J. 2008. Meta-analyses of cognitive functioning in euthymic bipolar patients and their first-degree relatives. *Psychol Med* **38**, 771–85.

Balanza-Martinez, V., Tabares-Seisdedos, R., Selva-Vera, G., *et al.* 2005. Persistent cognitive dysfunctions in bipolar I disorder and schizophrenic patients: a 3-year follow-up study. *Psychother Psychosom* **74**, 113–19.

Balanza-Martinez, V., Rubio, C., Selva-Vera, G., *et al.* 2008. Neurocognitive endophenotypes (endophenocognitypes) from studies of relatives of bipolar disorder subjects: a systematic review. *Neurosci Biobehav Rev* **32**, 1426–38.

Bell, M.D., Bryson, G.J., Greig, T.C., Fiszdon, J.M., & Wexler, B.E. 2005. Neurocognitive enhancement therapy with work therapy: productivity outcomes at 6- and 12-month follow-ups. *J Rehabil Res Dev* **42**, 829–38.

Berk, M., Hallam, K.T., & McGorry, P.D. 2007. The potential utility of a staging model as a course specifier: a bipolar disorder perspective. *J Affect Disord* **100**, 279–81.

Bonnín, C. del M., Martínez-Arán, A., Torrent, C., *et al.* 2010. Clinical and neurocognitive predictors of functional outcome in bipolar euthymic patients: a long-term, follow-up study. *J Affect Disord* **121**, 156–60.

Bonnín, C. del M., González-Pinto, A., Solé, B., *et al.*; CIBERSAM Functional Remediation Group. 2014. Verbal memory as a mediator in the relationship between subthreshold depressive symptoms and functional outcome in bipolar disorder. *J Affect Disord* **160**, 50–4.

Bora, E., Vahip, S., Akdeniz, F., *et al.* 2007. The effect of previous psychotic mood episodes on cognitive impairment in euthymic bipolar patients. *Bipolar Disord* **9**, 468–77.

Bora, E., Yucel, M., & Pantelis, C. 2009. Cognitive endophenotypes of bipolar disorder: a meta-analysis of neuropsychological deficits in euthymic patients and their first-degree relatives. *J Affect Disord* **113**, 1–20.

Bora, E., Yucel, M., & Pantelis, C. 2010. Neurocognitive markers of psychosis in bipolar disorder: a meta-analytic study. *J Affect Disord* **127**, 1–9.

Brenner, H.D., Hodel, B., Kienzle, N., Reed, D., & Liberman, R.P. 1994. *Integrated Psychological Therapy for Schizophrenic Patients*. Toronto: Hogrefe & Huber.

Broadbent, D.E. 1977. The hidden preattentive processes. *Am Psychol* **32**, 109–18.

Cannon, M., Caspi, A., Moffitt, T.E., *et al.* 2002. Evidence for early-childhood, pan-developmental impairment specific to schizophreniform disorder: results from a longitudinal birth cohort. *Arch Gen Psychiatry* **59**, 449–56.

Catalá-López, F., Gènova-Maleras, R., Alvarez-Martín, E., Fernández de Larrea-Baz, N., Morant-Ginestar, C. 2013. Burden of disease in adolescents and young people in Spain. *Rev Psiquiatr Salud Ment* **6**, 80–5.

Clark, L., Iversen, S.D., & Goodwin, G.M. 2002. Sustained attention deficit in bipolar disorder. *Br J Psychiatry* **180**, 313–19.

Colom, F. 2012. Social cognition and its potential role in bipolar disorder roughening: an editorial comment to Samamé C, Matino DJ, Strejilevich S. 'Social cognition in euthymic bipolar disorder: systematic review and meta-analytic approach'. *Acta Psychiatr Scand* **125**, 264–5.

Colom, F., Vieta, E., Martínez-Arán, A., *et al.* 2003. A randomized trial on the efficacy of group psychoeducation in the prophylaxis of recurrences in bipolar patients whose disease is in remission. *Arch Gen Psychiatry* **60**, 402–7.

Colom, F., Vieta, E., Daban, C., Pacchiarotti, I., & Sánchez-Moreno, J. 2006. Clinical and therapeutic implications of predominant polarity in bipolar disorder. *J Affect Disord* **93**, 13–17.

Coryell, W., Turvey, C., Endicott, J., *et al.* 1998. Bipolar I affective disorder: predictors of outcome after 15 years. *J Affect Disord* **50**, 109–16.

Daban, C., Colom, F., Sánchez-Moreno, J., Garcia-Amador, M., & Vieta, E. 2006a. Clinical correlates of first-episode polarity in bipolar disorder. *Compr Psychiatry* **47**, 433–7.

Daban, C., Martínez-Arán, A., Torrent, C., *et al.* 2006b. Cognitive functioning in bipolar patients receiving lamotrigine: preliminary results. *J Clin Psychopharmacol* **26**, 178–81.

Daban, C., Martínez-Arán, A., Torrent, C., *et al.* 2006c. Specificity of cognitive deficits in bipolar disorder versus schizophrenia: a systematic review. *Psychother Psychosom* **75**, 72–84.

Dean, B.B., Gerner, D., & Gerner, R.H. 2004. A systematic review evaluating health-related quality of life, work impairment, and healthcare costs and utilization in bipolar disorder. *Curr Med Res Opin* **20**, 139–54.

Deckersbach, T., Nierenberg, A.A., Kessler, R., *et al.* 2010. Cognitive rehabilitation for bipolar disorder: an open trial for employed patients with residual depressive symptoms. *CNS Neurosci Ther* **16**, 298–307.

Delahunty, A., & Morice, R. 1993. *The Frontal Executive Program. A Neurocognitive Rehabilitation Program for Schizophrenia*, revised edn. Albury, NSW, Australia: New South Wales Department of Health.

Delbello, M.P., Hanseman, D., Adler, C.M., Fleck, D.E., & Strakowski, S.M. 2007. Twelve-month outcome of adolescents with bipolar disorder following first hospitalization for a manic or mixed episode. *Am J Psychiatry* **164**, 582–90.

Demant, K.M., Almer, G.M., Vinberg, M., Kessing, L.V., & Miskowiak, K.W. 2013. Effects of cognitive remediation on cognitive dysfunction in partially or fully remitted patients with bipolar disorder. Study protocol for a randomized controlled trial. *Trials* **14**, 378. doi: 10.1186/1745-6215-14-378.

D'Zurilla, T.J., & Goldfried, M.R. 1971. Problem solving and behavior modification. *J Abnormal Psychol* **78**, 107–26.

Engelsmann, F., Katz, J., Ghadirian, A.M., & Schachter, D. 1988. Lithium and memory: a long-term follow-up study. *J Clin Psychopharmacol* **8**, 207–12.

Fagiolini, A., Kupfer, D.J., Masalehdan, A., *et al.* 2005. Functional impairment in the remission phase of bipolar disorder. *Bipolar Disord* **7**, 281–5.

Ferrier, I.N., & Thompson, J.M. 2002. Cognitive impairment in bipolar affective disorder: implications for the bipolar diathesis. *Br J Psychiatry* **180**, 293–5.

References

First, M.B., Spitzer, R., & Gibbon, M. 1997. *Structured Clinical Interview for DSM IV Axis I Disorder*, Research Version. New York, NY: Biometrics Research.

Fleck, D.E., Shear, P.K., Zimmerman, M.E., *et al.* 2003. Verbal memory in mania: effects of clinical state and task requirements. *Bipolar Disord* **5**, 375–80.

Frangou, S., Donaldson, S., Hadjulis, M., Landau, S., & Goldstein, L.H. 2005. The Maudsley Bipolar Disorder Project: executive dysfunction in bipolar disorder I and its clinical correlates. *Biol Psychiatry* **58**, 859–64.

Fuentes-Dura, I., Balanza-Martinez, V., Ruiz-Ruiz, J.C., *et al.* 2012. Neurocognitive training in patients with bipolar disorders: current status and perspectives. *Psychother Psychosom* **81**, 250–2.

Gitlin, M.J., Swendsen, J., Heller, T.L., & Hammen, C. 1995. Relapse and impairment in bipolar disorder. *Am J Psychiatry* **152**, 1635–40.

Glahn, D.C., Bearden, C.E., Niendam, T.A., & Escamilla, M.A. 2004. The feasibility of neuropsychological endophenotypes in the search for genes associated with bipolar affective disorder. *Bipolar Disord* **6**, 171–82.

Glahn, D.C., Bearden, C.E., Cakir, S., *et al.* 2006. Differential working memory impairment in bipolar disorder and schizophrenia: effects of lifetime history of psychosis. *Bipolar Disord* **8**, 117–23.

Glahn, D.C., Bearden, C.E., Barguil, M., *et al.* 2007. The neurocognitive signature of psychotic bipolar disorder. *Biol Psychiatry* **62**, 910–16.

Glahn, D.C., Almasy, L., Barguil, M., *et al.* 2010. Neurocognitive endophenotypes for bipolar disorder identified in multiplex multigenerational families. *Arch Gen Psychiatry* **67**, 168–77.

Goetz, I., Tohen, M., Reed, C., Lorenzo, M., & Vieta, E. 2007. Functional impairment in patients with mania: baseline results of the EMBLEM study. *Bipolar Disord* **9**, 45–52.

Goodwin, F.K., & Jamison, K.R. 2007. *Manic-Depressive Illness*, 2nd edn. New York, NY: Oxford University Press.

Gopin, C.B., Burdick, K.E., Derosse, P., Goldberg, T.E., & Malhotra, A.K. 2011. Emotional modulation of response inhibition in stable patients with bipolar I disorder: a comparison with healthy and schizophrenia subjects. *Bipolar Disord* **13**, 164–72.

Green, M.F., Kern, R.S., Braff, D.L., & Mintz, J. 2000. Neurocognitive deficits and functional outcome in schizophrenia: are we measuring the "right stuff"? *Schizophr Bull* **26**, 119–36.

Grynszpan, O., Perbal, S., Pelissolo, A., *et al.* 2011. Efficacy and specificity of computer-assisted cognitive remediation in schizophrenia: a meta-analytical study. *Psychol Med* **41**, 163–73.

Hammen, C., Gitlin, M., & Altshuler, L. 2000. Predictors of work adjustment in bipolar I patients: a naturalistic longitudinal follow-up. *J Consult Clin Psychol* **68**, 220–5.

Haro, J.M., Reed, C., Gonzalez-Pinto, A., *et al.* 2011. 2-year course of bipolar disorder type I patients in outpatient care: factors associated with remission and functional recovery. *Eur Neuropsychopharmacol* **21**, 287–93.

Hogarty, G.E., & Flesher, S. 1999a. Developmental theory for a cognitive enhancement therapy of schizophrenia. *Schizophr Bull* **25**, 677–92.

Hogarty, G.E., & Flesher, S. 1999b. Practice principles of cognitive enhancement therapy for schizophrenia. *Schizophr Bull* **25**, 693–708.

Hogarty, G.E., & Greenwald, D.P. 2006. *Cognititve Enhancment Therapy: The Training Manual*. Pittsburgh, PA: Western Psychiatric Institute and Clinic.

Huxley, N., & Baldessarini, R.J. 2007. Disability and its treatment in bipolar disorder patients. *Bipolar Disord* **9**, 183–96.

Judd, L.L., Akiskal, H.S., Schettler, P.J., *et al.* 2005. Psychosocial disability in the course of bipolar I and II disorders: a prospective, comparative, longitudinal study. *Arch Gen Psychiatry* **62**, 1322–30.

Judd, L.L., Schettler, P.J., Akiskal, H.S., *et al.* 2008. Residual symptom recovery from major affective episodes in bipolar disorders and rapid episode relapse/recurrence. *Arch Gen Psychiatry* **65**, 386–94.

Kanheman D. 1973. *Attention and Effort*. Englewood Cliffs, NJ: Prentice-Hall.

Kapczinski, F., Frey, B.N., Andreazza, A.C., *et al.* 2008a. Increased oxidative stress as a mechanism for decreased BDNF levels in acute manic episodes. *Rev Bras Psiquiatr* **30**, 243–5.

Kapczinski, F., Vieta, E., Andreazza, A.C., *et al.* 2008b. Allostatic load in bipolar disorder: implications for pathophysiology and treatment. *Neurosci Biobehav Rev* **32**, 675–92.

Keck, P.E., McElroy, S.L., Strakowski, S.M., *et al.* 1998. 12-month outcome of patients with bipolar disorder following hospitalization for a manic or mixed episode. *Am J Psychiatry* **155**, 646–52.

Keefe, R.S., Vinogradov, S., Medalia, A., *et al.* 2011. Report from the working group conference on multisite trial design for cognitive remediation in schizophrenia. *Schizophr Bull* **37**, 1057–65.

Kessler, R.C., Akiskal, H.S., Ames, M., *et al.* 2006. Prevalence and effects of mood disorders on work performance in a nationally representative sample of U.S. workers. *Am J Psychiatry* **163**, 1561–8.

Kolur, U.S., Reddy, Y.C., John, J.P., Kandavel, T., & Jain, S. 2006. Sustained attention and executive functions in euthymic young people with bipolar disorder. *Br J Psychiatry* **189**, 453–58.

Krabbendam, L., & Aleman, A. 2003. Meta-analyses of randomized controlled trials of social skills training and cognitive remediation. *Psychol Med* **33**, 756–8.

Kronhaus, D.M., Lawrence, N.S., Williams, A.M., *et al.* 2006. Stroop performance in bipolar disorder: further evidence for abnormalities in the ventral prefrontal cortex. *Bipolar Disord* **8**, 28–39.

Kurtz, M.M., Moberg, P.J., Gur, R.C., & Gur, R.E. 2001. Approaches to cognitive remediation of neuropsychological deficits in schizophrenia: a review and meta-analysis. *Neuropsychol Rev* **11**, 197–210.

Lezak, M.D., Howieson, D.B., Loring, D.B., Hannay, H.J., & Fisher, J.S. 2004. *Neuropsychological Assessment*, 4th edn. New York, NY: Oxford University Press.

López-Jaramillo, C., Lopera-Vásquez, J., Gallo, A., *et al.* 2010a. Effects of recurrence on the cognitive performance of patients with bipolar I disorder: implications for relapse prevention and treatment adherence. *Bipolar Disord* **12**, 557–67.

López-Jaramillo, C., Lopera-Vásquez, J., Ospina-Duque, J., *et al.* 2010b. Lithium treatment effects on the neuropsychological functioning of patients with bipolar I disorder. *J Clin Psychiatry* **71**, 1055–60.

Luria, A.R. 1963. *Restoration of Function after Brain Injury*. New York, NY: Pergamon Press.

MacQueen, G.M., Young, L.T., Robb, J.C., *et al.* 2000. Effect of number of episodes on wellbeing and functioning of patients with bipolar disorder. *Acta Psychiatr Scand* **101**, 374–81.

MacQueen, G.M., Young, L.T., & Joffe, R.T. 2001. A review of psychosocial outcome in patients with bipolar disorder. *Acta Psychiatr Scand* **103**, 163–70.

Malhi, G.S., Ivanovski, B., Hadzi-Pavlovic, D., *et al.* 2007. Neuropsychological deficits and functional impairment in bipolar depression, hypomania and euthymia. *Bipolar Disord* **9**, 114–25.

Martínez-Arán, A., Vieta, E., Colom, F., *et al.* 2000. Cognitive dysfunctions in bipolar disorder: evidence of neuropsychological disturbances. *Psychother Psychosom* **69**, 2–18.

Martínez-Arán, A., Vieta, E., Colom, F., *et al.* 2004a. Cognitive impairment in euthymic bipolar patients: implications for clinical and functional outcome. *Bipolar Disord* **6**, 224–32.

Martínez-Arán, A., Vieta, E., Reinares, M., *et al.* 2004b. Cognitive function across manic or hypomanic, depressed, and euthymic states in bipolar disorder. *Am J Psychiatry* **161**, 262–70.

Martínez-Arán, A., Vieta, E., Torrent, C., *et al.* 2007. Functional outcome in bipolar disorder: the role of clinical and cognitive factors. *Bipolar Disord* **9**, 103–13.

Martínez-Arán, A., Torrent, C., Tabares-Seisdedos, R., *et al.* 2008. Neurocognitive impairment in bipolar patients with and without history of psychosis. *J Clin Psychiatry* **69**, 233–9.

Martínez-Arán, A., Torrent, C., Sole, B., *et al.* 2011. Functional remediation for bipolar disorder. *Clin Pract Epidemiol Ment Health* **7**, 112–16.

Martino, D.J., Marengo, E., Igoa, A., *et al.* 2009. Neurocognitive and symptomatic predictors of functional outcome in bipolar disorders: a prospective 1 year follow-up study. *J Affect Disord* **116**, 37–42.

McEwen, B.S., & Stellar, E. 1993. Stress and the individual: mechanisms leading to disease. *Arch Intern Med* **153**, 2093–101.

McGurk, S.R., Twamley, E.W., Sitzer, D.I., McHugo, G.J., & Mueser, K.T. 2007. A meta-analysis of cognitive remediation in schizophrenia. *Am J Psychiatry* **164**, 1791–802.

Medalia, A., & Choi, J. 2009. Cognitive remediation in schizophrenia. *Neuropsychol Rev* **19**, 353–64.

Medalia, A., & Herlands, T. 2002. *Remediation of Cognitive Deficits in Psychiatric Outpatients: A Clinician's Manual*. New York, NY: Montefiore Medical Center Press.

Medalia, A., Revheim, N., & Casey, M. 2002. Remediation of problem-solving skills in schizophrenia: evidence of a persistent effect. *Schizophr Res* **57**, 165–71.

Moritz, S., & Woodward, T.S. 2005. *Metacognitive Skill Training for Patients with Schizophrenia (MCT)*. Hamburg: VanHam Campus Press.

Muñoz Cespedes, J.M., & Tirapu Ustarroz, J. 2001. *Rehabilitación Neuropsicológica*. Madrid: Sintesis.

Mur, M., Portella, M.J., Martínez-Arán, A., Pifarré, J., & Vieta, E. 2008. Neuropsychological profile in bipolar disorder: a preliminary study of monotherapy lithium-treated euthymic bipolar patients evaluated at a 2-year interval. *Acta Psychiatr Scand* **118**, 373–81.

Murray, C.J., & Lopez, A.D. 1997. Global mortality, disability, and the contribution of risk factors: Global Burden of Disease Study. *Lancet* **349**, 1436–42.

Parker, G., Rosen, A., Trauer, T., & Hadzi-Pavlovic, D. 2007. Disability associated with mood states and comparator conditions: application of the Life Skills Profile measure of disability. *Bipolar Disord* **9**, 11–15.

Penadés, R., & Gastó, C. 2010. *El Tratamiento de Rehabilitación Neurocognitiva en la Esquizofrenia*. Barcelona: Herder Editorial.

Penadés, R., & Boget, T. 1999. *No Me Acuerdo: Trastornos de la Memoria*. Editorial Océano.

Penadés, R., Boget, T., Salamero, M., Catarineu, S., & Bernardo, M. 1999. [Neuropsychological alteration in schizophrenia and its modification]. *Actas Esp Psiquiatr* **27**, 198–208.

Pilling, S., Bebbington, P., Kuipers, E., *et al.* 2002. Psychological treatments in schizophrenia: II. Meta-analyses of randomized controlled trials of social skills training and cognitive remediation. *Psychol Med* **32**, 783–91.

Pomarol-Clotet, E., Moro, N., Sarro, S., *et al.* 2012. Failure of de-activation in the medial frontal cortex in mania: evidence for default mode network dysfunction in the disorder. *World J Biol Psychiatry* **13**, 616–26.

Preiss, M., Shatil, E., Cermáková, R., Cimermanová, D., & Ram, I. 2013. Personalized cognitive training in unipolar and bipolar disorder: a study of cognitive functioning. *Front Hum Neurosci* **7**, 108. doi: 10.3389/fnhum.2013.00108.

Prigatano, G.P. 1999. *Principles of Neuropsychological Rehabilitation*. New York, NY: Oxford University Press.

Reichenberg, A., Weiser, M., Rabinowitz, J., *et al*. 2002. A population-based cohort study of premorbid intellectual, language, and behavioral functioning in patients with schizophrenia, schizoaffective disorder, and nonpsychotic bipolar disorder. *Am J Psychiatry* **159**, 2027–35.

Robinson, L.J., & Ferrier, I.N. 2006. Evolution of cognitive impairment in bipolar disorder: a systematic review of cross-sectional evidence. *Bipolar Disord* **8**, 103–16.

Rosa, A.R., Sánchez-Moreno, J., Martínez-Arán, A., *et al*. 2007. Validity and reliability of the Functioning Assessment Short Test (FAST) in bipolar disorder. *Clin Pract Epidemol Ment Health* **3**, 5.

Rosa, A.R., Franco, C., Martínez-Arán, A., *et al*. 2008. Functional impairment in patients with remitted bipolar disorder. *Psychother Psychosom* **77**, 390–2.

Rosa, A.R., Bonnín, C.M., Mazzarini, L., *et al*. 2009. Predictores clínicos del funcionamiento interpersonal en pacientes bipolares. *Rev Psiquiatr Salud Ment (Barc)* **2**, 83–8.

Rosa, A.R., Reinares, M., Amann, B., *et al*. 2011. Six-month functional outcome of a bipolar disorder cohort in the context of a specialized-care program. *Bipolar Disord* **13**, 679–86.

Rougier, N.P., Noelle, D.C., Braver, T.S., Cohen, J.D., & O'Reilly, R.C. 2005. Prefrontal cortex and flexible cognitive control: rules without symbols. *Proc Natl Acad Sci U S A* **102**, 7338–43.

Ruggero, C.J., Chelminski, I., Young, D., & Zimmerman, M. 2007. Psychosocial impairment associated with bipolar II disorder. *J Affect Disord* **104**, 53–60.

Samamé, C., Martino, D.J., & Strejilevich, S.A. 2012. Social cognition in euthymic bipolar disorder: systematic review and meta-analytic approach. *Acta Psychiatr Scand* **125**, 266–80.

Sánchez-Moreno, J., Martínez-Arán, A., Colom, F., *et al*. 2009a. Neurocognitive dysfunctions in euthymic bipolar patients with and without prior history of alcohol use. *J Clin Psychiatry* **70**, 1120–7.

Sánchez-Moreno, J., Martínez-Arán, A., Tabares-Seisdedos, R., *et al*. 2009b. Functioning and disability in bipolar disorder: an extensive review. *Psychother Psychosom* **78**, 285–97.

Simon, G.E., Ludman, E.J., Unutzer, J., Operskalski, B.H., & Bauer, M.S. 2008. Severity of mood symptoms and work productivity in people treated for bipolar disorder. *Bipolar Disord* **10**, 718–25.

Smith, M.J. 1975. *When I Say No, I Feel Guilty: How to Cope, Using the Skills of Systematic Assertive Therapy*. New York, NY: Dial Press.

Sohlberg, M., Johnson, L., Paule, L., Raskin, S., & Mateer, C.A. 1994. *Attention Process Training II: A Program to Address Attentional Deficits for Persons with Mild Cognitive Dysfunction*. Puyallup, WA: Association for Neuropsychological Research and Development.

Sole, B., Bonnín, C.M., Torrent, C., *et al*. 2012. Neurocognitive impairment and psychosocial functioning in bipolar II disorder. *Acta Psychiatr Scand* **125**, 309–17.

Spreen, O., & Strauss, E. 1998. *A Compendium of Neuropsychological Tests: Administration, Norms, and Commentary*, 2nd edn. New York, NY: Oxford University Press.

Strakowski, S.M., Keck, P.E., Jr., McElroy, S.L., *et al*. 1998. Twelve-month outcome after a first hospitalization for affective psychosis. *Arch Gen Psychiatry* **55**, 49–55.

Strakowski, S.M., Williams, J.R., Fleck, D.E., & Delbello, M.P. 2000. Eight-month functional outcome from mania following a first psychiatric hospitalization. *J Psychiatr Res* **34**, 193–200.

Tabares-Seisdedos, R., Escamez, T., Martinez-Gimenez, J.A., *et al*. 2006. Variations in genes regulating neuronal migration predict reduced prefrontal cognition in schizophrenia and bipolar subjects from Mediterranean Spain: a preliminary study. *Neuroscience* **139**, 1289–300.

Thompson, J.M., Gallagher, P., Hughes, J.H., *et al.* 2005. Neurocognitive impairment in euthymic patients with bipolar affective disorder. *Br J Psychiatry* **186**, 32–40.

Tohen, M., Hennen, J., Zarate, C.M., *et al.* 2000. Two-year syndromal and functional recovery in 219 cases of first-episode major affective disorder with psychotic features. *Am J Psychiatry* **157**, 220–8.

Tohen, M., Greil, W., Calabrese, J.R., *et al.* 2005. Olanzapine versus lithium in the maintenance treatment of bipolar disorder: a 12-month, randomized, double-blind, controlled clinical trial. *Am J Psychiatry* **162**, 1281–90.

Tohen, M., Bowden, C.L., Calabrese, J.R., *et al.* 2006. Influence of sub-syndromal symptoms after remission from manic or mixed episodes. *Br J Psychiatry* **189**, 515–19.

Tohen, M., Vieta, E., Gonzalez-Pinto, A., Reed, C., & Lin, D. 2010. Baseline characteristics and outcomes in patients with first episode or multiple episodes of acute mania. *J Clin Psychiatry* **71**, 255–61.

Torrent, C., Martínez-Arán, A., Daban, C., *et al.* 2006. Cognitive impairment in bipolar II disorder. *Br J Psychiatry* **189**, 254–9.

Torrent, C., Martínez-Arán, A., Amann, B., *et al.* 2007. Cognitive impairment in schizoaffective disorder: a comparison with non-psychotic bipolar and healthy subjects. *Acta Psychiatr Scand* **116**, 453–60.

Torrent, C., Martínez-Arán, A., Del Mar, B.C., *et al.* 2012. Long-term outcome of cognitive impairment in bipolar disorder. *J Clin Psychiatry* **73**, e899–905.

Torrent, C., Bonnín, C.M., Martínez-Arán, A., *et al.* 2013. Efficacy of functional remediation in bipolar disorder: a multicenter randomized controlled study. *Am J Psychiatr* **170**, 852–9.

Torres, I.J., Boudreau, V.G., & Yatham, L.N. 2007. Neuropsychological functioning in euthymic bipolar disorder: a meta-analysis. *Acta Psychiatr Scand Suppl* (434), 17–26.

Torres, I.J., DeFreitas, V.G., DeFreitas, C.M., *et al.* 2010. Neurocognitive functioning in patients with bipolar I disorder recently recovered from a first manic episode. *J Clin Psychiatry* **71**, 1234–42.

Tremont, G., & Stern, R.A. 1997. Use of thyroid hormone to diminish the cognitive side effects of psychiatric treatment. *Psychopharmacol Bull* **33**, 273–80.

Tremont, G., & Stern, R.A. 2000. Minimizing the cognitive effects of lithium therapy and electroconvulsive therapy using thyroid hormone. *Int J Neuropsychopharmacol* **3**, 175–86.

Twamley, E.W., Jeste, D.V., & Bellack, A.S. 2003. A review of cognitive training in schizophrenia. *Schizophr Bull* **29**, 359–82.

van Gorp, W.G., Altshuler, L., Theberge, D.C., Wilkins, J., & Dixon, W. 1998. Cognitive impairment in euthymic bipolar patients with and without prior alcohol dependence: a preliminary study. *Arch Gen Psychiatry* **55**, 41–6.

Vargas, M., & Jimeno, N. 2002. *Esquizofrneia e Insuficiencia Atencional*. Valladolid: Universidad de Valladolid.

Vieta, E., & Gasto, C. 1997. *Trastornos Bipolares*. Barcelona: Springer-Verlag Iberica.

Vieta, E., Popovic, D., Rosa, A.R., *et al.* 2013. The clinical implications of cognitive impairment and allostatic load in bipolar disorder. *Eur Psychiatry* **28**, 21–9.

Vinogradov, S., Fisher, M., & de Villers-Sidani, E. 2012. Cognitive training for impaired neural systems in neuropsychiatric illness. *Neuropsychopharmacology* **37**, 43–76.

Wykes, T., & Reeder, C. 2005. *Cognitive Remediation Therapy: Theory and Practice*. Hove: Routledge.

Wykes, T., & Spaulding, W.D. 2011. Thinking about the future cognitive remediation therapy–what works and could we do better? *Schizophr Bull* **37** Suppl 2, S80–90.

Yan, L.J., Hammen, C., Cohen, A.N., Daley, S.E., & Henry, R.M. 2004. Expressed emotion versus relationship quality variables in the prediction of recurrence in bipolar patients. *J Affect Disord* **83**, 199–206.

Zammit, S., Allebeck, P., David, A.S., *et al.* 2004. A longitudinal study of premorbid IQ Score and risk of developing schizophrenia, bipolar disorder, severe depression, and other nonaffective psychoses. *Arch Gen Psychiatry* **61**, 354–60.

Zarate, C.A., Tohen, M., Land, M., & Cavanagh, S. 2000. Functional impairment and cognition in bipolar disorder. *Psychiatr Q* **71**, 309–29.

Index